Senior's Diabetic Cookbook for Beginners

1800+ Days of Mouthwatering Low-Carb, Low-Sugar Recipes for Pre-Diabetes and Type 2 Diabetes in Later Years | Healthier, Independent Living with 30-Day Plan

by

Ingrid Lamarr

Dear Reader,

We wish to share with you an essential decision we've made regarding the editions of our books, a choice driven by our commitment to sustainability and the preservation of our planet.

We have chosen to print the physical copies of our books in **black and white**. This decision has been made with deep reflection and awareness based on various key reasons related to environmental sustainability:

- **Ink Saving**: Black and white printing uses less ink, and the production of black ink is generally less environmentally impactful than colored ink.
- **Energy Efficiency**: Printers for black-and-white production consume less energy than color printers.
- **Waste Reduction**: We can reduce waste generated from expended cartridges by minimizing the use of multiple ink cartridges.
- **Lower Costs**: Reduced black-and-white printing costs allow for more economical and accessible production, with less environmental impact from production and distribution.
- **Sustainable Material Use**: We commit to using recycled paper or paper from sustainable sources alongside eco-friendly printing practices.

We acknowledge that some of you might prefer to enjoy our books in their vibrant and colorful entirety. For this reason, **each physical copy of our book will contain an exclusive QR code** allowing you to access a **digital, colored version** of the book. This will provide you with the opportunity to experience the content in a colorful format and read the book across various electronic devices, enhancing your reading experience.

We recognize the value and importance of your experience as a reader and want to ensure that, even as we adopt measures to be more eco-friendly and sustainable, you do not miss out on the wondrous world enclosed within the pages of our books.

Thank you for your ongoing support and understanding regarding this decision. Your passion for reading and commitment to a more sustainable future makes this community special.

With gratitude and commitment towards a greener future,

Ingrid Lamarr

Lend Us Your Voice in Our Journey

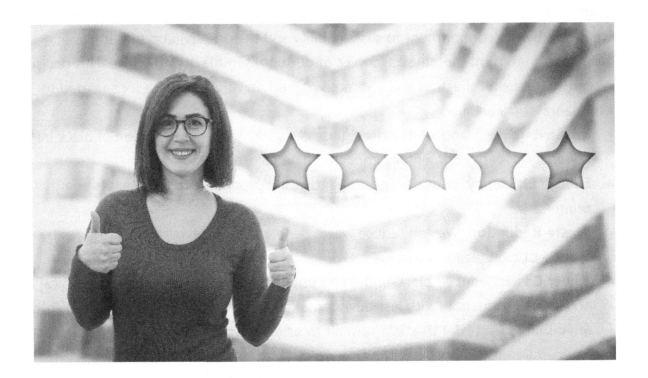

As a publisher, every single review is fundamental support for us. Your voice can make a difference and help us continue our mission. If you believe in the value of what we do and want to lend us a hand, please take a moment to share your thoughts.

Your review is our beacon in the vast sea of publishing. From the bottom of our hearts, thank you for your invaluable contribution!

http://bit.ly/diabeticrev

GET YOUR BONUSES NOW!

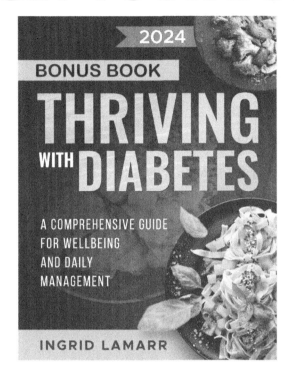
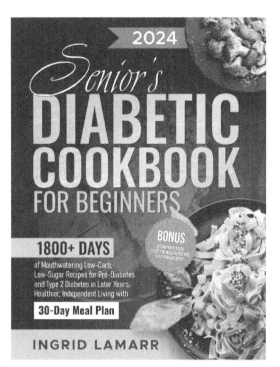

Download your FREE BONUSES now!

Go to the Bonus page and download this amazing FREE BONUS.

TABLE OF CONTENTS

Sommario

INTRODUCTION: NOURISHING THE BODY AND SOUL

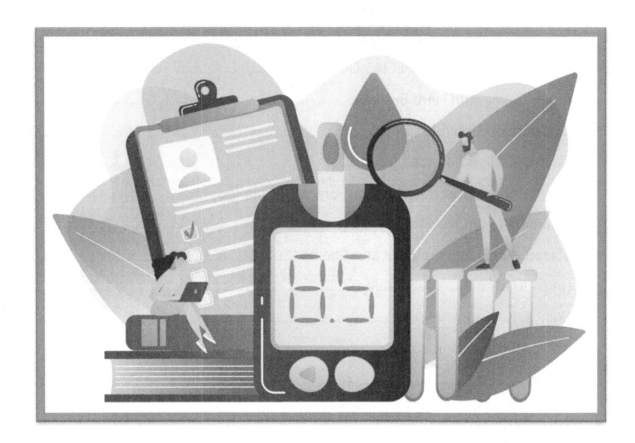

MY PERSONAL STORY

I have always heard about the sickness of diabetes, but I have never taken the time to learn so much about it. I have been to the hospital and seen so many people with these health conditions, but I have not been so close to sharing in their pains until a very close friend of mine was diagnosed with this health condition.

At first, I didn't know how to react, what to tell her, or what to do! I could see her facial reaction. It was as if she was in deep pain. I consoled her and told her to take things easy. When she had calmed down a bit, the doctor began to speak. He told her that someone with diabetes could still live in good health if the condition is properly managed. He also advised her not to allow herself to be stressed out.

When we left the hospital, I knew I had to look for every means possible to help my friend reduce the pain she must be feeling and also the fear she has of not being able to live a normal life again. The various research I did led me to write this book.

COOKBOOK OBJECTIVE

In this cookbook, we tackle the challenge of diabetes with a practical approach. The condition can be overwhelming, but this guide simplifies daily tasks and makes them understandable, debunking the myth that healthy eating is synonymous with bland and unfulfilling meals.

Included are delicious, easy-to-prepare, and affordable recipes that focus on healthy eating for everyone. Covering everything from breakfast to dinner, including snacks and desserts, this book offers a comprehensive range of meals that cater to the dietary needs of those with diabetes and those seeking enjoyable, flavorful dishes. Discover valuable insights into managing diabetes effectively through diet, ensuring you never have to compromise on taste or variety.

BRIEF OVERVIEW OF TYPE 2 DIABETES

Type 2 diabetes, a common condition, occurs when blood sugar levels increase. The body uses blood glucose for energy, mainly from food. Insulin, a hormone the pancreas produces, helps cells absorb glucose for energy. In type 2 diabetes, the body either makes too little insulin or doesn't use it effectively, leading to excess sugar in the blood and not enough in the cells.

Type 2 diabetes is no respecter of age, even in infancy. However, middle-aged and older individuals are more commonly affected by this type of diabetes. Risk factors include obesity, a family history of diabetes, and being over 45. African Americans, Hispanics/Latinos, American Indians, Asian Americans, and Pacific Islanders are also more likely to have diabetes.

Various factors can cause type 2 diabetes, some of which are hypertension and a lack of physical activity. Also, if you have once had prediabetes or had gestational diabetes while you were pregnant, then type 2 diabetes is possible. Symptoms include increased thirst and urination, hunger, fatigue, blurred vision, numbness in extremities, non-healing sores, and unexplained weight loss.

Sometimes, you might easily notice you have this condition because it can be a minor sign, and it frequently develops gradually over the years. Many people don't exhibit any signs. Some people might not be aware of the condition until they experience certain complications like heart disease or cloudy eyesight.

Various factors are responsible for it, which includes;
- Overweight and obesity

- Not being physically active
- Insulin resistance
- genes

Important strategies to deal with this condition include controlling blood pressure, cholesterol, and blood sugar levels; if you smoke, you should also stop. Diabetes management includes lifestyle changes like eating nutritious meals, reducing calorie intake if overweight, and regular physical activity.

There might be a need for you to have diabetes medications like pills or subcutaneous injections of insulin in addition to complying with your diabetes care plan. You might need more than one diabetic medication over time to manage your blood sugar effectively. Even if you don't take insulin, there are situations when you could need it, like when you're pregnant or when you're in the hospital. Additionally, you could require medication for illnesses like hypertension, high cholesterol, or others

CHAPTER 1: UNDERSTANDING NUTRITION IN DIABETES

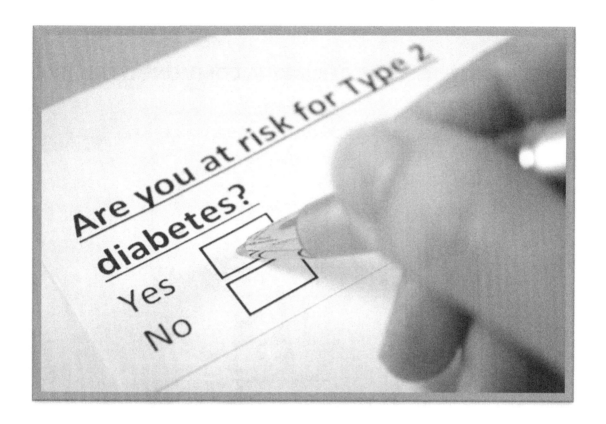

This chapter explores nutrition's crucial role in managing Type 2 Diabetes. We will debunk common myths, understand the impact of macronutrients on blood sugar, learn about portion control, and emphasize the importance of blood sugar monitoring.

For some years, certain data from observational research and clinical attempts have been brought together to support the role of various nutrients and foods in preventing and controlling type 2 diabetes.

The quality of dietary fats and carbohydrates eaten is much more important than the quantity of these macronutrients. Diets that can minimize diabetes risk and boost glycemic control and blood lipids include:

- fruits
- vegetables
- nuts
- moderate alcohol use
- high whole grains
- low refined grains

- red/processed meats
- legumes, etc.

MYTHS VS. REALITY: BEGIN BY DEBUNKING COMMON MYTHS ABOUT DIABETES.

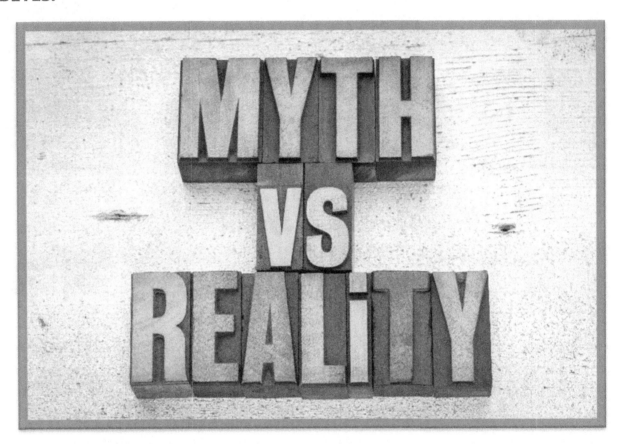

Diabetes can be described as a chronic disease in which the body cannot regulate the amount of glucose in the blood. This disease is quite difficult to comprehend. If you have this disease or you know of someone who does, you may have certain questions about it you would like to have answered. There are various prevalent misconceptions regarding this disease and its care. In the section below, we will take a look at some of them;

Myth: My relative doesn't have the disease; hence, I won't.
Fact: It's quite true that when you have a relative who has this disease, you are also at greater risk of having the disease. Family history is a huge risk factor for type 2 diabetes, yet so many diabetic individuals cannot blame heredity for it. Choices of lifestyle and some conditions can result in type 2 diabetes. Some of these choices include being obese or overweight, being above forty-five, Being

Hispanic/Latino, African American, American Indian, or Alaska Native (certain Pacific Islanders and Asian Americans are also at risk).

Myth: I take so much sugar, and this is making me worry that I might have diabetes.
Fact: The fact that you love to take sugary substances doesn't mean you will have diabetes. However, you must reduce the sweets and sugary beverages you take.
I understand when people are seriously concerned about how they consume sugary substances. This might be because they know that when they consume food, it is transformed into sugar, known as glucose. Glucose (blood sugar) is a type of energy the body uses. Insulin sends glucose from the bloodstream into cells to utilize it as energy. Even though this is true, there is no need to panic if you consume a lot of sugar.

Having dispelled these myths, let's delve deeper into the scientific realities of diabetes nutrition, starting with the fundamental role of macronutrients.

NUTRITION FUNDAMENTALS: INTRODUCTION TO MACRONUTRIENTS AND HOW THEY AFFECT BLOOD SUGAR.

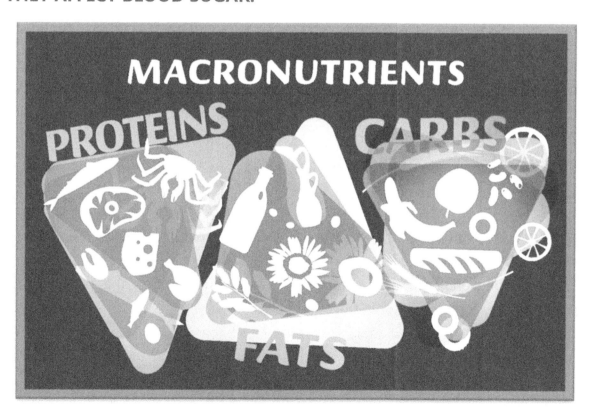

When the term nutrition is being discussed, two types readily come to one's mind: macronutrients and micronutrients. Macronutrients are nutrients that people need in large quantities and regularly to provide energy to their bodies so that they will have enough strength to carry out their daily activities.

Most of the time, macronutrients are proteins, carbs, and fats; there are also times when some people will choose to add other nutrients that others also require in high quantities, such as water. Macronutrients produce most of the energy and calories used by the body. Each macronutrient contains advantages and functions in keeping a healthy body. Individual factors like weight, age, and other underlying health issues can also affect how much of each macronutrient an individual needs.

The primary sugar in the body, blood glucose, which can also be referred to as blood sugar, is the body's major energy source. You can get it from your diet. Most of what you consume is usually transformed into glucose by your body and then released into your bloodstream. Anytime your blood glucose levels rise, your pancreas will send a signal for insulin to be released. Insulin is a hormone for transporting glucose into cells for use as energy.

To control your blood sugar, you need to pay close attention to the carbohydrate element of your diet. Proteins are not so important to us. Although you can also turn them into blood sugar, it can only happen when there is enough protein, and it does this very slowly and inefficiently. Lastly, fat is the only macronutrient that does not convert to sugar and produces the least amount of insulin. When taken into the body, carbohydrates are disintegrated into simple sugar molecules and then enter the bloodstream as they are digested. Due to this, blood glucose and insulin levels will rise. Consuming a potato, a slice of bread, or a cake has the same effect: they raise blood sugar quickly because they are carbs.

For your breakfast, lunch, or even dinner, as well as snacks throughout the day, eating carb items helps you maintain your glucose and insulin levels. When your cells receive high insulin levels for an extended period, they become less responsive. With this, there might be insulin resistance. With a clear understanding of macronutrients, we now turn to practical applications in daily eating, beginning with managing food portions effectively.

PORTION GUIDE: EXPLANATION OF PORTIONS AND FOOD GROUPS.

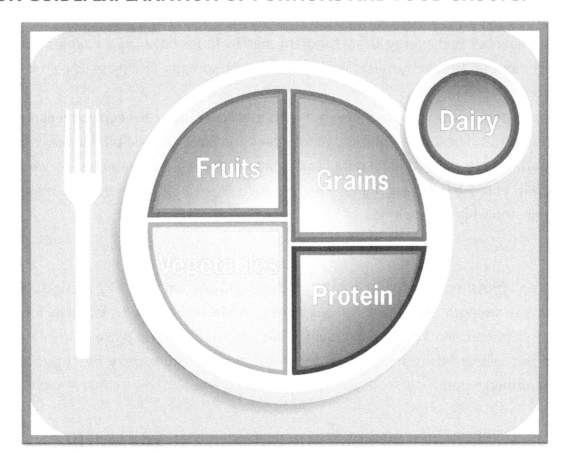

There are five food groups in our world today: fruit and vegetables, starchy food, Dairy, protein, and fat. In the section below, you will learn more about these food groups and how much you need to eat.

Fruit and vegetables

Fruits and vegetables have much to offer you, so eating at least portions daily isn't bad. Fruit and veggies have relevant vitamins and minerals to prevent disease and fiber that can help reduce cholesterol for a good bowel and help ease digestion.

Fruits and veggies are quite low in fat; hence, they are nice and satisfy you without adding too many calories.

Examples of a portion of fruit and vegetables include;
- One apple, banana, pear, orange, or some other fruit the same size as the ones mentioned.
- Half a grapefruit or avocado
- One slice of a big fruit like watermelon or pineapple.

Starchy food

One-third of your food should have potatoes, bread, rice, and pasta. They are rich in vitamins, calcium, iron, essential fiber, and energy. Gram for gram, starchy foods have fewer calories than fat. Steer clear of adding more fat to starchy meals like jam, butter, oil, spreads, or cheese since this will increase the calorie count.

Wholegrain foods are typically higher in nutrients and fiber. They can keep you feeling fuller for longer since you cannot digest them quickly. Wholegrain breakfast cereals, brown rice, wholewheat pasta, whole oats, whole meal bread, pitta, and chapatti are a few examples of whole grain foods. Additionally, you can purchase higher-fiber products like 50/50 bread that are manufactured with a wholegrain and white flour blend.

Dairy

Vitamins and protein can be found in dairy products and alternatives. They also include calcium, which supports the strength and health of our bones. While having lower fat than full-fat milk, semi-skimmed, skimmed, and 1% fat milk provides calcium, vitamins, and protein.

Soy and nut milk are dairy-free substitutes; if you decide to use dairy-free milk, choose the plain, calcium-fortified types.

Fat

While some fat is necessary in our meals, most consume too much. As a highly unsaturated fat, plant-based oils like olive, rapeseed, and vegetable oil minimize cholesterol and heart disease. Butter can be substituted with lower-fat unsaturated spreads.

Chocolate, cakes, biscuits, savory snacks, and drinks contain excess fat, salt, or sugar. This type of food accounts for half of Scotland's sugar intake and about 20% of its calories and fat. Foods and beverages with so much fat, salt, and sugar are usually said to have a high-calorie content and little nutritional value; thus, they shouldn't be included in a balanced, healthful diet.

Protein: Pulses

When you need to add some stuff to food like meat sauces, soups, and casseroles, you can also use pulses, which are very good for things like that. When you use pulses, you can use less meat because they help increase the flavor and texture. Once that is done, less fat will be consumed, and it also ensures that your money goes further because pulses are less expensive than meat.

Another very good example of a protein that you can consider is egg. There is no suggestion of limiting the quantity of eggs you can consume weekly, and they make a nutritious meal. You can make use of eggs for preparing fast, healthful meals. When cooking eggs, try limiting the amount of fat you add. It is best if you boil, scramble, or poach. If you decide to fry eggs, use healthy and unsaturated oils, including vegetable, rapeseed, or olive oil, and don't add too much to the pan.

BLOOD SUGAR MONITORING: THE IMPORTANCE OF MONITORING AND HOW TO DO IT CORRECTLY

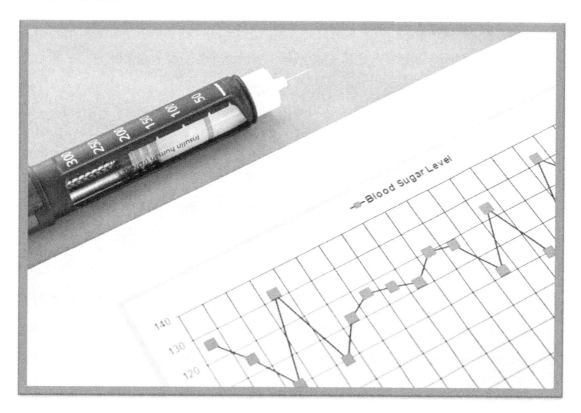

If you have diabetes, always ensure that you regularly check your blood sugar because that is how you will get to know if your drug is working well or not. It will guide you on how to take care of your diabetes daily and even hourly. Checking your blood sugar regularly is very important if you have diabetes and especially if you are using insulin. The results you will get from your examination determine what you should eat and how much you should eat. You can also learn how much exercise and insulin you should take.

There are so many factors that can have an impact on your blood sugar. Some of these effects are very difficult or impossible to foresee, but as time goes on and with experience, you should be able to know some of them. If your healthcare practitioner asks that you check your blood sugar frequently, ensure that you do so.

There are two ways you can check your blood sugar in the comfort of your home if you have diabetes;

- Using a glucose meter and finger stick.

- A continuous glucose monitor (CGM) is a 24-hour glucose monitoring device that must be worn before using CGM. Using this information, the device will make a graph that provides a more comprehensive view of the fluctuations in your blood sugar.
  - Wash your hands. For example, food particles on your fingers may have affected the outcome of your test. If soap and water are unavailable, wipe your fingertips with alcohol.
  - Take a test strip and place it in your glucose meter.
  - A drop of blood is what you need. Just puncture the side of the tip of your finger with the use of a lancing tool. If you can't get enough blood, you might need to prick or squeeze a new finger more.
  - When you have done the above and await your results, touch the test strip's edge and hold on to it. The screen of the meter will then show your blood glucose level.

FAQ: FREQUENTLY ASKED QUESTIONS ABOUT TYPE 2 DIABETIC NUTRITION.

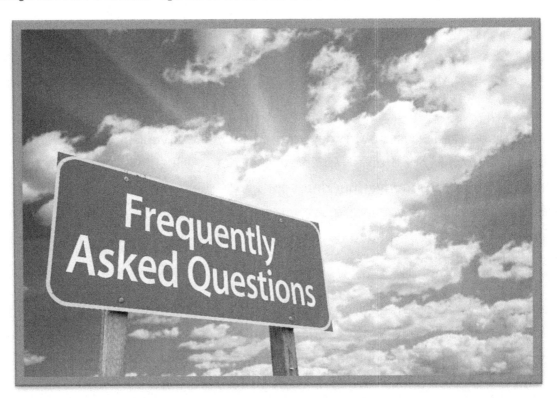

What foods are both type 2 diabetes-friendly and help your heart?

It can be difficult to think of a diet that benefits cardiovascular and diabetic health. The truth is that to take preventive measures against cardiovascular disease (CVD) by managing your diabetes, you may be eating a healthy diet to make that possible.

- **Are there any diets I should go on or any I should avoid?**

There is no need for you to believe what people are saying about going on a diet if you have type 2 diabetes and you are at risk for heart disease. There's a bad thought to this kind of thinking, and most diets fail or go away on their own.

Ensure that you do not start a diet you know you might be unable to comply with completely. Think about your main objectives, which include having stable blood sugar, a positive report concerning your heart from your physician, and total control of your well-being with better vigor for life, rather than the various foods you cannot eat.

- **Why is it important to reduce carbs and sugar in your diet?**

While they are not the ones you are against, carbohydrates are very important and a healthy component of a balanced diet. However, individuals with type 2 diabetes who eat enough refined grains, sugary drinks, and desserts should be thinking about reducing the amount of carbohydrates they consume.

Choose diverse complex carbs with much higher fiber content, a range of vitamins, and some other nutrients. Because fiber reduces the rate at which sugar gets into the system, it is very good for diabetic people. In the end, this will help in the regulation of blood glucose.

In conclusion, this chapter has interconnected the myths, realities, nutritional fundamentals, portion guidance, and the importance of blood sugar monitoring, offering a comprehensive view on managing Type 2 Diabetes through informed dietary choices.

CHAPTER 2: THE PERFECT BREAKFAST

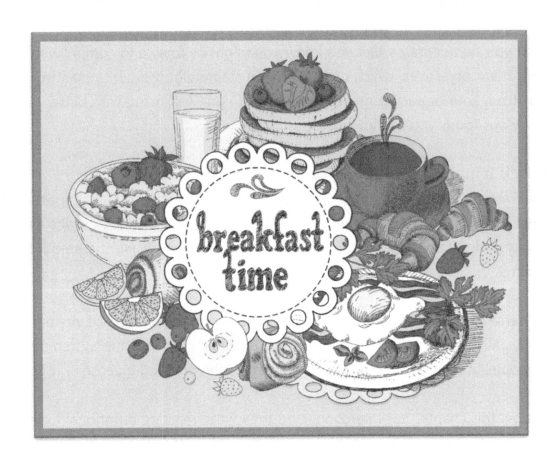

RECIPES: PROVIDE SEVERAL BREAKFAST OPTIONS THAT ARE BALANCED AND NUTRITIOUS.

Starting your day with a nutritious breakfast is not only recommended for maintaining overall health but also plays a role in reducing the risk of certain health issues. Research suggests that skipping breakfast may be linked to an increased likelihood of being overweight and may impact overall diet quality. Those who skip this essential meal often miss crucial nutrients and might consume more calories and added sugars later in the day. Breakfast helps stabilize blood sugar levels and can keep you energized and less likely to feel hungry frequently. It's particularly important for children, as a balanced breakfast aids in improving concentration and building lean muscles through protein and low-fat dairy, while carbohydrates rich in minerals and fiber support their overall growth and development.

Despite some debate, the consensus in the health sector leans towards breakfast being an important meal. It's crucial to ensure your breakfast is nutritious, incorporating a balance of high-fiber carbohydrates, healthy fats, and proteins. High-fiber foods, such as fruits, vegetables, oats, and whole wheat, help moderate blood sugar spikes and sustain energy levels. Proteins and fats contribute to feeling full, assisting in better daily hunger management.

Oatmeal with Berries and Nuts

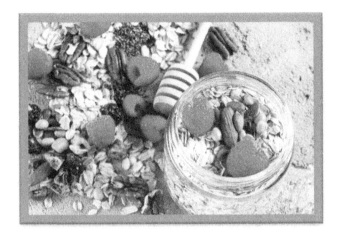

Recipe Description

This heart-healthy oatmeal breakfast contains fiber, antioxidants, and omega-3 fatty acids. Combining whole-grain oats, fresh berries, and nuts provides a balanced meal to start the day, perfect for seniors managing Type 2 diabetes.

Preparation Time: 15 min

Cooking Time: 5 min

Servings: 4

Glycemic Index: Low

Ingredients:

- 1 cup rolled oats
- 2 cups water
- Pinch of salt
- 1 cup mixed berries (blueberries, strawberries, raspberries)
- 1/4 cup chopped nuts (almonds, walnuts)
- 2 tablespoons ground flaxseed
- Stevia or Erythritol to taste (optional)

Directions

1. **Prepare the Water:** Bring 2 cups of water to a boil in a medium saucepan. Add a pinch of salt to the water – this will enhance the flavor of the oats.

2. **Cook the Oats:** Add 1 cup of rolled oats once the water is boiling. Reduce the heat to a simmer. Let the oats cook for about 5 minutes, stirring occasionally to prevent sticking. The oats should absorb the water and become soft yet retain a bit of chew.

3. **Divide the Oatmeal:** Remove the saucepan from the heat after the oats are cooked. Divide the oatmeal evenly into four serving bowls. This will be the base for your toppings.

4. **Add Toppings:** Evenly distribute the mixed berries on top of the hot oatmeal. You can combine blueberries, strawberries, and raspberries for various flavors and textures. Then, sprinkle each bowl with the chopped nuts of your choice, such as almonds or walnuts, for a crunchy texture and healthy fats.

5. **Include Ground Flaxseed:** Add a half tablespoon of ground flaxseed to each bowl. Flaxseed is a great omega-3 fatty acids and fiber source, adding nutritional value to your meal.

6. **Sweeten if Desired:** If you prefer a sweeter taste, sweeten each bowl of oatmeal with a natural sweetener like Stevia or Erythritol. Adjust the amount to suit your taste preference.

7. **Serve:** Stir each bowl of oatmeal to mix the toppings in well and enjoy a hearty, nutritious breakfast.

Nutritional Values (per serving)

- Calories: 150

- Protein: 6g
- Carbohydrates: 23g
- Fat: 7g
- Fiber: 5g
- Sodium: 40mg

Macronutrient Breakdown
- Protein: 16%
- Carbohydrates: 61%
- Fat: 23%

Recipe Tips:
- Using organic berries and nuts can provide the best nutritional and anti-inflammatory benefits.
- Ground flaxseeds add omega-3 fatty acids that benefit heart health and enhance texture.

Allergy Alert:
- Contains nuts. For a nut-free version, substitute nuts with pumpkin or sunflower seeds.

Substitutions for Vegans: No substitutions are needed.

Substitutions for Gluten Intolerance: Ensure oats are certified gluten-free.

Scrambled Eggs with Spinach and Whole Wheat Toast

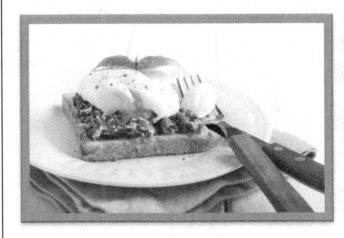

Recipe Description

This classic and nutritious American breakfast combines fluffy scrambled eggs with iron-rich spinach, served with whole wheat toast. It's an easy and quick meal, perfect for seniors looking to start their day with a protein-rich, diabetic-friendly option.

Preparation Time: 10 min

Cooking Time: 5 min

Servings: 4

Glycemic Index: Low

Ingredients:
- 8 large eggs
- 2 cups fresh spinach, chopped
- 4 slices of whole wheat bread
- 1 tablespoon olive oil
- Salt and pepper to taste

Directions

1. **Whisk the Eggs:** In a large bowl, break the eggs and whisk them together with a pinch of salt and pepper. Ensure the eggs are well-beaten to incorporate air, which makes the scrambled eggs fluffy.
2. **Prepare the Spinach:** Rinse the fresh spinach and chop it roughly. Chopping

the spinach helps it blend easily with the eggs and cook more evenly.

3. **Cook the Spinach:** Heat a tablespoon of olive oil in a non-stick skillet over medium heat. Once the oil is hot, add the chopped spinach to the skillet. Sauté the spinach for 1-2 minutes or until it wilts. Stir continuously to prevent the spinach from sticking to the pan.

4. **Scramble the Eggs:** Pour the whisked eggs over the wilted spinach in the skillet. Let the eggs sit briefly before stirring, then gently stir with a spatula. Cook for 2-3 minutes, stirring occasionally, until the eggs are cooked but moist. Avoid overcooking to keep the texture soft and creamy.

5. **Toast the Bread:** While the eggs cook, toast the whole wheat bread slices in a toaster until golden brown and crisp.

6. **Serve the Dish:** Remove the skillet from the heat once the eggs are cooked to your liking. Serve the scrambled eggs immediately, accompanied by the toasted whole wheat bread.

Nutritional Values (per serving)

- Calories: 250, Protein: 19g, Carbohydrates: 16g, Fat: 13g, Fiber: 3g, Sodium: 400mg

Macronutrient Breakdown

- Protein: 30%
- Carbohydrates: 26%
- Fat: 44%

Recipe Tips:

- Using organic eggs and spinach can provide additional health benefits.

- Whole wheat toast adds fiber to the meal, making it more balanced and filling.

Allergy Alert:

- Contains eggs and wheat. For a gluten-free option, substitute with gluten-free bread.

Substitutions for Vegans: Replace eggs with a tofu scramble.

Substitutions for Gluten Intolerance: Use gluten-free bread.

Greek Yogurt with Mixed Berries and Nuts

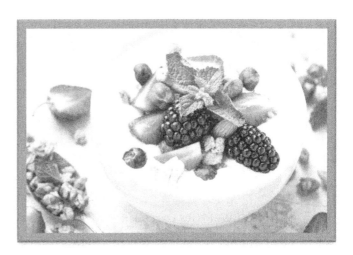

Recipe Description

This refreshing and easy-to-prepare breakfast features Greek yogurt with a medley of berries and nuts. It's a delightful combination of protein, healthy fats, and antioxidants, making it a superb choice for seniors managing Type 2 diabetes.

Preparation Time: 5 min

Cooking Time: 0 min

Servings: 4

Glycemic Index: Low

Ingredients:

- 2 cups Greek yogurt, low-fat

- 1 cup mixed berries (blueberries, raspberries, strawberries)
- 1/4 cup mixed nuts (almonds, walnuts), chopped
- 1 tablespoon chia seeds
- Stevia or Erythritol to taste (optional)

Directions

1. **Prepare the Serving Bowls:** Begin by taking four serving bowls. Divide the Greek yogurt evenly among the bowls. Greek yogurt serves as a high-protein, creamy base for the toppings.
2. **Wash and Prepare Berries:** Gently wash the mixed berries - blueberries, raspberries, and strawberries. If the strawberries are large, slice them into smaller pieces. Evenly distribute the berries on top of the yogurt in each bowl, adding various colors and flavors.
3. **Add Nuts and Chia Seeds:** Chop the mixed nuts if not already chopped. Sprinkle a mixture of chopped almonds and walnuts over the yogurt and berries in each bowl for a crunchy texture. Then, add a sprinkle of chia seeds to each bowl. Chia seeds are a great source of fiber and omega-3 fatty acids.
4. **Optional Sweetening:** If desired, sweeten each serving with Stevia or Erythritol. Adjust the amount according to your taste preference, especially considering dietary needs for managing diabetes.
5. **Serve the Dish:** The Greek yogurt bowls are ready to serve once all the toppings are added. This dish is best enjoyed fresh.

Nutritional Values (per serving)

- Calories: 180, Protein: 12g, Carbohydrates: 15g, Fat: 8g, Fiber: 3g, Sodium: 50mg

Macronutrient Breakdown

- Protein: 27%
- Carbohydrates: 33%
- Fat: 40%

Recipe Tips:

- Using organic berries and nuts can enhance the health benefits of the meal.
- Chia seeds add nutritional value and a pleasant texture to the yogurt.

Allergy Alert:

- Contains dairy and nuts. For a dairy-free version, substitute with almond or soy yogurt.

Substitutions for Vegans: Use plant-based yogurt such as almond, soy, or coconut yogurt.

Substitutions for Gluten Intolerance: No substitutions are needed; the recipe is gluten-free.

Apple Cinnamon Oatmeal Pancakes

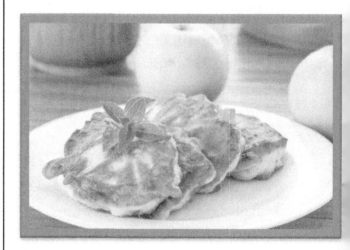

Recipe Description

These Apple Cinnamon offer a delicious twist on a traditional breakfast. Made with wholesome

Ingredients: like oats and fresh apples, they are perfect for seniors looking for a hearty, low-glycemic breakfast.

Preparation Time: 20 min

Cooking Time: 10 min

Servings: 4

Glycemic Index: Low

Ingredients:

- 1 cup rolled oats
- 1 medium apple, grated
- 2 large eggs
- 1/2 cup almond milk
- 1 tsp cinnamon
- 1 tsp baking powder
- Olive oil or cooking spray (for cooking)
- Sugar-free syrup or honey (optional for serving)

Directions

1. **Create Oat Flour:** Start by placing rolled oats in a blender. Blend until they reach a fine, flour-like consistency. This oat flour will be the base of your pancake batter.

2. **Prepare the Batter:** In a mixing bowl, combine the freshly made oat flour, grated apple, eggs, almond milk, cinnamon, and baking powder. Stir the mixture until all **Ingredients:** are well incorporated, and you have a smooth batter. The grated apple adds natural sweetness and moisture.

3. **Heat the Pan:** Place a non-stick pan over medium heat. Lightly coat the pan with olive oil or cooking spray to prevent the pancakes from sticking.

4. **Cook the Pancakes:** Pour about 1/4 cup of batter for each pancake onto the hot pan. Cook the pancakes until bubbles form on the surface, usually taking 2-3 minutes. Then, carefully flip each pancake and cook the other side until golden brown, which should take another 2-3 minutes.

5. **Serving:** Once the pancakes are cooked, serve them hot. You can top them with sugar-free syrup or a drizzle of honey for added sweetness.

Nutritional Values (per serving)

Calories: 180, Protein: 6g, Carbohydrates: 27g, Fat: 6g, Fiber: 4g, Sodium: 150mg

Macronutrient Breakdown

Protein: 13%, Carbohydrates: 60%, Fat: 27%

Recipe Tips:

- Using a non-stick pan is crucial for easy flipping and to keep the pancakes from tearing apart.
- The grated apple in the batter adds natural sweetness and moistens the pancakes.

Allergy Alert:

- Contains eggs. Use a flax egg (1 tbsp ground flaxseed mixed with 2.5 tbsp water) for an egg-free version.

Substitutions for Vegans: Replace eggs with flax eggs.

Substitutions for Gluten Intolerance: Ensure oats are certified gluten-free.

Turkey and Vegetable Frittata

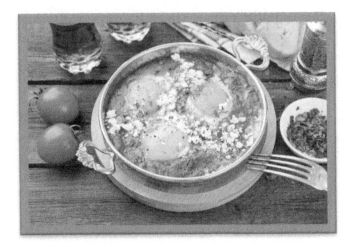

Recipe Description

This Turkey and Vegetable Frittata is a perfect blend of lean protein and fresh vegetables, making it an ideal breakfast for seniors. It's a versatile dish that can be enjoyed hot or cold and is diabetic-friendly and nutritious.

Preparation Time: 15 min

Cooking Time: 20 min

Servings: 4

Glycemic Index: Low

Ingredients:

- 6 large eggs
- 1/2 cup cooked turkey breast, diced
- 1 cup spinach, chopped
- 1/2 cup bell peppers, diced
- 1/4 cup onions, chopped
- 1/4 cup low-fat cheese, shredded
- 1 tbsp olive oil
- Salt and pepper to taste

Directions

1. **Preheat the Oven:** Preheat your oven to 375°F (190°C). This temperature is suitable for cooking the frittata evenly.
2. **Whisk the Eggs:** In a large bowl, break the eggs and whisk them together. Season with a pinch of salt and pepper. This forms the base of your frittata.
3. **Prepare the Vegetables:** Wash and chop the spinach, dice the bell peppers, and chop the onions. These vegetables will add flavor and nutrients to the frittata.
4. **Cook the Vegetables and Turkey:** Heat olive oil in an oven-safe skillet over medium heat. Add the onions, bell peppers, and spinach to the skillet. Sauté until the vegetables are soft, about 3-5 minutes. Add the diced cooked turkey to the skillet and stir to combine.
5. **Add the Egg Mixture:** Pour the seasoned egg mixture over the cooked vegetables and turkey in the skillet. Make sure the eggs are evenly distributed.
6. **Add Cheese:** Sprinkle the shredded low-fat cheese over the top of the egg mixture. This will melt and create a delicious topping.
7. **Bake the Frittata:** Transfer the skillet to the preheated oven. Bake for 15-20 minutes or until the eggs are set and the top is lightly golden.
8. **Serving:** Once done, remove the frittata from the oven. Let it cool for a few minutes, then slice and serve warm.

Nutritional Values (per serving)

Calories: 220, Protein: 20g, Carbohydrates: 6g, Fat: 13g, Fiber: 1g, Sodium: 320mg

Macronutrient Breakdown

Protein: 36%, Carbohydrates: 11%, Fat: 53%

Recipe Tips:

- Feel free to customize this frittata with any vegetables you have on hand for additional flavors and nutrients.

- If you prefer a vegetarian version, you can omit the turkey or substitute it with chicken or another protein source.

Allergy Alert:
- Contains eggs and dairy. For a dairy-free version, omit the cheese.

Substitutions for Vegans: Use a tofu scramble instead of eggs and skip the cheese.

Substitutions for Gluten Intolerance: No substitutions are needed; the recipe is gluten-free.

Banana Walnut Baked Oatmeal

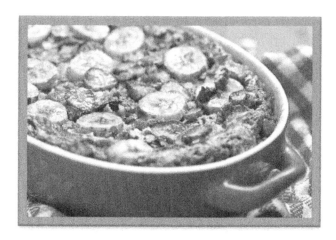

Recipe Description

This Banana Walnut Baked Oatmeal offers a warm, comforting, and nutritious start to the day. It's a great diabetic-friendly breakfast option for seniors, combining the natural sweetness of bananas with the heartiness of oats and the crunch of walnuts.

Preparation Time: 10 min

Cooking Time: 25 min

Servings: 4

Glycemic Index: Low

Ingredients:
- 2 cups rolled oats
- 1 ripe banana, mashed
- 1/4 cup walnuts, chopped
- 2 cups almond milk
- 1 tsp vanilla extract
- 1 tsp cinnamon
- 1 tbsp honey or sugar-free syrup (optional)
- Cooking spray for greasing

Directions
1. **Preheat the Oven:** Preheat your oven to 350°F (175°C). This temperature is ideal for baking oatmeal to a perfect consistency.
2. **Prepare the Baking Dish:** Grease a medium-sized baking dish with cooking spray. This prevents the oatmeal from sticking to the dish.
3. **Mix the Ingredients::** In a large bowl, combine the rolled oats, mashed ripe banana, and chopped walnuts. The banana should be overripe for added natural sweetness. Add almond milk, vanilla extract, and cinnamon to the bowl. Stir the mixture until all the **Ingredients:** are well combined.
4. **Pour into Baking Dish:** Transfer the oatmeal mixture into the greased baking dish. Spread it evenly with a spoon or spatula.
5. **Bake the Oatmeal:** Place the baking dish in the preheated oven. Bake for about 25 minutes, or until the top of the oatmeal is golden and the oats are set.
6. **Optional Sweetening:** After baking, you can drizzle the top of the baked oatmeal

with honey or sugar-free syrup for added sweetness, if desired.

7. **Serving:** Remove the baked oatmeal from the oven. Let it cool slightly, then serve it warm.

Nutritional Values (per serving)

Calories: 240, Protein: 8g, Carbohydrates: 38g, Fat: 7g, Fiber: 6g, Sodium: 80mg

Macronutrient Breakdown

Protein: 13%, Carbohydrates: 63%, Fat: 24%

Recipe Tips:

- Use overripe bananas for their natural sweetness and moisture.
- This dish can be prepared ahead of time and reheated for a convenient and quick breakfast.

Allergy Alert:

- Contains nuts. For a nut-free version, omit the walnuts or replace them with pumpkin or sunflower seeds.

Substitutions for Vegans: No substitutions are needed; the recipe is already vegan.

Substitutions for Gluten Intolerance: Ensure oats are certified gluten-free.

Avocado Toast with Poached Eggs

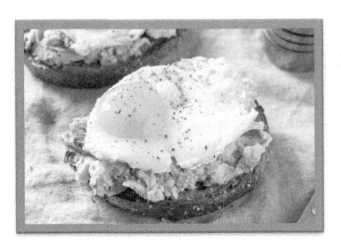

Recipe Description

This modern twist on a classic breakfast, Avocado Toast with Poached Eggs, is delicious, heart-healthy, and diabetic-friendly. It's a great option for seniors, combining the creamy texture of avocado with the protein-rich goodness of eggs, all served on whole-grain toast.

Preparation Time: 15 min

Cooking Time: 10 min

Servings: 4

Glycemic Index: Low

Ingredients:

- 4 slices whole wheat bread
- 2 ripe avocados
- 4 large eggs
- 1 tbsp white vinegar
- Salt and pepper to taste
- Red pepper flakes (optional)

Directions

1. **Toast the Bread:** Begin by toasting the whole wheat bread slices in a toaster or the oven until golden brown and crispy.
2. **Prepare the Avocado Spread:** Cut the avocados in half, remove the pits, and

scoop the flesh into a bowl. Mash the avocado with a fork until it reaches a creamy consistency. Season the mashed avocado with salt and pepper to taste.

3. **Spread Avocado on Toast:** Evenly spread the mashed avocado onto the toasted bread slices. The avocado spread will be the base for the poached eggs.

4. **Poach the Eggs:** Fill a pot with about 3 inches of water and bring it to a simmer. Add a tablespoon of white vinegar to the water. Crack each egg into a small cup or bowl and carefully slide them into the simmering water. Cook the eggs for 3-4 minutes for soft, runny yolks or a little longer if you prefer firmer yolks. Use a slotted spoon to remove the eggs from the water.

5. **Assemble the Avocado Toast:** Place a poached egg on top of each slice of avocado toast. The egg should sit neatly on the avocado spread.

6. **Add Seasoning:** Season each avocado toast with a pinch of salt, pepper, and red pepper flakes if desired for added spice.

Nutritional Values (per serving)
Calories: 300, Protein: 12g, Carbohydrates: 20g, Fat: 20g, Fiber: 7g, Sodium: 200mg
Macronutrient Breakdown
Protein: 16%, Carbohydrates: 27%, Fat: 57%

Recipe Tips:
- Use ripe avocados for the best flavor and creamy texture.
- Depending on your preference or dietary needs, you can replace poached eggs with scrambled or fried ones.

Allergy Alert:

- Contains wheat and eggs. For a gluten-free option, use gluten-free bread.

Substitutions for Vegans: Replace eggs with a tofu scramble or sliced tomatoes for a vegan version.

Substitutions for Gluten Intolerance: Use gluten-free bread.

Berry Smoothie Bowl

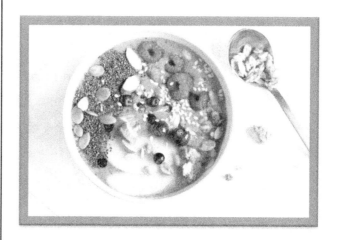

Recipe Description
This Berry Smoothie Bowl is a visually appealing breakfast and nutritious, diabetic-friendly option for seniors. It blends a variety of berries for a high antioxidant kick, combined with the creamy texture of Greek yogurt, perfect for a refreshing start to the day.

Preparation Time: 10 min
Cooking Time: 0 min
Servings: 4
Glycemic Index: Low

Ingredients:
- 2 cups mixed berries (blueberries, strawberries, raspberries)
- 2 cups Greek yogurt, low-fat
- 1/4 cup almond milk

- 1 tbsp chia seeds
- 1 tbsp honey or sugar-free syrup (optional)
- Additional berries and nuts for topping

Directions

1. **Blend the Smoothie Mixture:** In a blender, combine 2 cups of mixed berries (you can use fresh or frozen berries for a thicker consistency), 2 cups of low-fat Greek yogurt, and 1/4 cup of almond milk. Blend these **Ingredients:** until the mixture is smooth and creamy.
2. **Pour into Bowls:** Distribute the smoothie mixture evenly into four serving bowls.
3. **Add Toppings:** Sprinkle 1 tablespoon of chia seeds over each bowl. Chia seeds add fiber and omega-3 fatty acids to the meal. Then, add additional berries on top for extra flavor and nutrients. You can also add various nuts for added crunch and healthy fats.
4. **Sweeten if Desired:** If you prefer a sweeter taste, drizzle each bowl with a tablespoon of honey or sugar-free syrup.
5. **Serve Immediately:** Enjoy the berry smoothie bowl immediately while it's fresh and cold.

Nutritional Values (per serving)
Calories: 150, Protein: 10g, Carbohydrates: 18g, Fat: 4g, Fiber: 3g, Sodium: 50mg
Macronutrient Breakdown
Protein: 27%, Carbohydrates: 48%, Fat: 25%

Recipe Tips:

- Using frozen berries will give the smoothie bowl a thicker and more refreshing texture.
- Customize your smoothie bowl with your favorite nuts and seeds for extra texture and nutrients.

Allergy Alert:

- Contains dairy. For a dairy-free version, substitute with plant-based yogurt.

Substitutions for Vegans: Use plant-based yogurt instead of Greek yogurt.

Substitutions for Gluten Intolerance: No substitutions are needed; the recipe is gluten-free.

Vegetable and Cheese Omelette

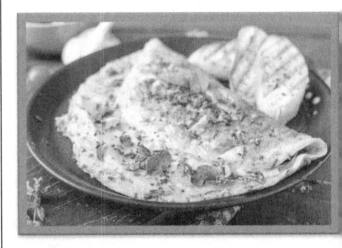

Recipe Description

A Vegetable and Cheese Omelette is a nutritious and satisfying breakfast for seniors. This dish is rich in protein and packed with various vegetables, making it a great choice for a diabetic-friendly meal.

Preparation Time: 10 min
Cooking Time: 10 min
Servings: 4
Glycemic Index: Low

Ingredients:

- 8 large eggs

- 1 cup mixed vegetables (bell peppers, spinach, mushrooms)
- 1/2 cup low-fat cheese, shredded
- 1 tbsp olive oil
- Salt and pepper to taste

Directions

1. **Beat the Eggs:** In a large bowl, crack the eggs and beat them until well combined. Season with salt and pepper to enhance the flavor.
2. **Prepare the Vegetables:** Chop the bell peppers, spinach, and mushrooms into small, bite-sized pieces. This allows them to cook evenly and mix well with the eggs.
3. **Sauté the Vegetables:** Heat the olive oil in a non-stick skillet over medium heat. Add the chopped vegetables to the skillet and sauté them until they are soft about 3-5 minutes. Stir occasionally to ensure even cooking.
4. **Cook the Omelette:** Pour the beaten eggs over the sautéed vegetables in the skillet, ensuring the eggs spread evenly. Allow the eggs to cook undisturbed for a few minutes until they start to set.
5. **Add Cheese:** Sprinkle the shredded low-fat cheese over the eggs. The cheese will melt as the omelet cooks, adding a creamy texture.
6. **Finish Cooking:** Continue cooking until the eggs are fully set. Once the bottom is cooked and the top is just about set, carefully fold the omelet in half with a spatula, enclosing the vegetables and cheese.
7. **Serve:** Slide the omelet onto a plate and serve it hot. You can cut it into portions if desired.

Nutritional Values (per serving)

Calories: 230, Protein: 20g, Carbohydrates: 5g, Fat: 15g, Fiber: 1g, Sodium: 320mg

Macronutrient Breakdown

Protein: 35%, Carbohydrates: 9%, Fat: 56%

Recipe Tips:

- Incorporate a variety of colorful vegetables to enhance the nutrient content.
- You can customize the omelet with your preferred vegetables or cheese.

Allergy Alert:

- Contains eggs and dairy. For a dairy-free version, omit the cheese.

Substitutions for Vegans: Use a chickpea flour batter instead of eggs and skip the cheese.

Substitutions for Gluten Intolerance: No substitutions are needed; the recipe is gluten-free.

Whole Wheat Blueberry Muffins

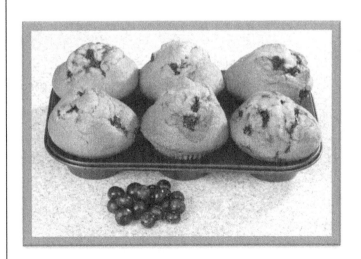

Recipe Description

These Whole Wheat Blueberry Muffins are a delightful and nutritious breakfast for seniors. Made with whole wheat flour and fresh blueberries, they are a great source of fiber and antioxidants, making them suitable for a diabetic-friendly diet.

Preparation Time: 15 min

Cooking Time: 20 min

Servings: 4 (2 muffins per serving)

Glycemic Index: Low

Ingredients:

- 1 1/2 cups whole wheat flour
- 3/4 cup fresh blueberries
- 1/2 cup unsweetened applesauce
- 1/4 cup honey or sugar-free syrup
- 2 large eggs
- 1/2 cup low-fat milk
- 1 tsp baking powder
- 1/2 tsp baking soda
- 1/2 tsp vanilla extract
- Pinch of salt

Directions

1. **Preheat the Oven:** Preheat your oven to 375°F (190°C). Prepare a muffin tin with paper liners or grease it with cooking spray. This prevents the muffins from sticking.
2. **Mix Dry Ingredients::** In a large mixing bowl, combine the whole wheat flour, baking powder, baking soda, and a pinch of salt. Stir these **Ingredients:** together to distribute the leavening agents evenly.
3. **Whisk Wet Ingredients::** In a separate bowl, whisk together the eggs, unsweetened applesauce, honey (or sugar-free syrup), low-fat milk, and vanilla extract. Ensure these **Ingredients:** are well combined.
4. **Combine Wet and Dry Ingredients::** Gently fold the wet and dry **Ingredients:**. Mix until combined to avoid overworking the batter, making the muffins tough.
5. **Add Blueberries:** Carefully stir the fresh blueberries into the batter. Fresh blueberries are recommended for the best flavor and nutrient content.
6. **Fill Muffin Tin:** Spoon the batter into the prepared muffin tin, filling each cup about 3/4 full. This allows room for the muffins to rise without overflowing.
7. **Bake:** Place the muffin tin in the oven for 20 minutes. Check for doneness by inserting a toothpick into the center of a muffin; it should come out clean.
8. **Cool and Serve:** Remove the muffin tin from the oven once baked. Allow the muffins to cool in the tin for a few minutes, then transfer them to a wire rack to cool completely.

Nutritional Values (per serving)

Calories: 220, Protein: 6g, Carbohydrates: 40g, Fat: 4g, Fiber: 5g, Sodium: 200mg

Macronutrient Breakdown

Protein: 11%, Carbohydrates: 73%, Fat: 16%

Recipe Tips:

- Using fresh blueberries will enhance the muffins' flavor and nutritional value.
- These muffins can be stored in an airtight container, making them a convenient breakfast option throughout the week.

Allergy Alert:

- Contains wheat and eggs. For a gluten-free version, substitute with gluten-free flour.

Substitutions for Vegans: Replace eggs with flax eggs (1 tbsp ground flaxseed mixed with 2.5 tbsp water per egg) and milk with almond milk.

Substitutions for Gluten Intolerance: Use gluten-free flour.

CHAPTER 3: LIGHT AND TASTY LUNCHES

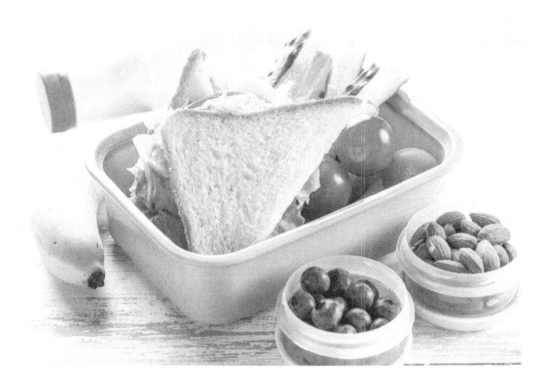

Lunch can be challenging to eat healthily, but with a little preparation and forethought, you can make it the highlight of your day. As these delicious recipes demonstrate, there are plenty more creative, healthy lunch alternatives than just a dull bed of greens. Even though some of these require a bit more work, the majority of these may be prepared in 15 minutes or less. A few recipes can also be prepared beforehand, so you can prepare them tonight and arrange them before dinner.

Nutrient-dense foods like proteins and vegetables are a staple of many of our favorite lunch recipes and your belly will still be accommodating them until dinnertime. Consider wholesome chicken and salmon recipes, delectable dairy products like yogurt and cottage cheese, and garnishes like nutritional yeast and sunflower seeds.

Furthermore, don't be shocked if you see a lot of high-fiber items like chickpeas and avocados, which both offer a ton of sustained energy and a full stomach; therefore, whether you're searching for satisfying and delectable low-calorie meals, nutritious sandwiches, salads, or a crispy, fresh flatbread pizza. After all, eating well shouldn't ever feel restrictive.

Tuna Salad with Whole Wheat Pita

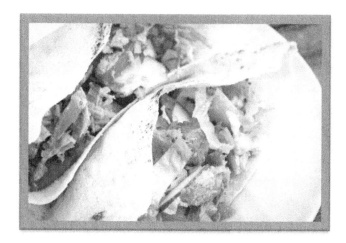

Recipe Description

This Tuna Salad with Whole Wheat Pita is a classic American lunch, ideal for seniors. It's light, nutritious, and easy to prepare, combining the lean protein of tuna with the wholesomeness of whole wheat pita bread.

Preparation Time: 10 min

Cooking Time: 0 min

Servings: 4

Glycemic Index: Low

Ingredients:

- 2 cans of tuna in water, drained
- 1/4 cup low-fat mayonnaise
- 1 celery stalk, finely chopped
- 1 small onion, finely chopped
- 1/2 teaspoon black pepper
- 4 whole wheat pita bread halves
- Lettuce leaves

Directions

1. **Prepare the Tuna Salad:** In a medium-sized bowl, combine the drained tuna, low-fat mayonnaise, finely chopped celery, and finely chopped onion. Season the mixture with black pepper. Mix thoroughly until the tuna is well coated with mayonnaise and the vegetables are evenly distributed.
2. **Assemble the Pita:** Take the whole wheat pita bread halves and gently open them to create pockets. Be careful not to tear the bread.
3. **Stuff the Pita with Tuna Salad:** Spoon equal amounts of the tuna salad into each pita bread half. The salad should be evenly distributed among the pita halves.
4. **Add Lettuce:** Insert a few leaves into each pita pocket on the tuna salad. The lettuce adds extra crunch and nutrition to the meal.
5. **Serving:** Serve the tuna salad and stuffed pita breads immediately. They are best enjoyed fresh.

Nutritional Values (per serving)

Calories: 200, Protein: 20g, Carbohydrates: 20g, Fat: 6g, Fiber: 3g, Sodium: 300mg

Macronutrient Breakdown

Protein: 40%, Carbohydrates: 40%, Fat: 20%

Recipe Tips:

- Opt for canned tuna in water instead of oil-packed for a healthier choice.
- Add a squeeze of fresh lemon juice to the tuna salad for added freshness and a hint of citrus flavor.

Allergy Alert:

- Contains fish and wheat. For a gluten-free option, use gluten-free pita bread.

Substitutions for Vegans: Replace the tuna with a chickpea salad mixture.

Substitutions for Gluten Intolerance: Use gluten-free pita bread.

Chicken and Avocado Lettuce Wraps

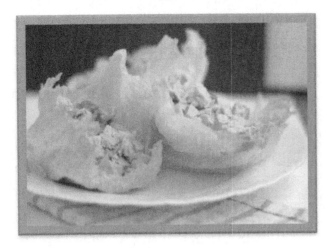

Recipe Description

Chicken and Avocado Lettuce Wraps are a light, healthy lunch option for seniors. This recipe features tender chicken and creamy avocado wrapped in crisp lettuce leaves, making it a delightful and diabetic-friendly choice.

Preparation Time: 15 min

Cooking Time: 0 min (if using pre-cooked chicken)

Servings: 4

Glycemic Index: Low

Ingredients:

- 2 cups cooked chicken breast, shredded
- 1 ripe avocado, diced
- 1/2 cup cherry tomatoes, halved
- 1/4 cup red onion, finely chopped
- 1 tablespoon lime juice
- 8 large lettuce leaves (e.g., Romaine or Butter lettuce)
- Salt and pepper to taste

Directions

1. **Prepare the Filling:** In a medium-sized bowl, combine the shredded cooked chicken breast, diced ripe avocado, halved cherry tomatoes, and finely chopped red onion.

2. **Season the Mixture:** Drizzle the tablespoon of lime juice over the chicken and avocado mixture. The lime juice adds flavor and helps prevent the avocado from browning. Season the mixture with salt and pepper to taste. Gently stir everything to ensure the **Ingredients:** are well mixed.

3. **Assemble the Wraps:** Lay out the lettuce leaves on a clean surface. Spoon an equal amount of the chicken and avocado mixture onto the center of each lettuce leaf.

4. **Wrap It Up:** Carefully fold the lettuce leaves around the filling, tucking in the edges to create a wrap. The lettuce should hold the filling snugly but be gentle to avoid tearing the leaves.

5. **Serving:** Serve the lettuce wraps immediately while fresh and crisp.

Nutritional Values (per serving)

Calories: 180, Protein: 18g, Carbohydrates: 8g, Fat: 10g, Fiber: 4g, Sodium: 60mg

Macronutrient Breakdown

Protein: 40%, Carbohydrates: 18%, Fat: 42%

Recipe Tips:

- Using pre-cooked chicken breast simplifies preparation and saves time.
- The addition of lime juice not only enhances flavor but also helps maintain the freshness of the avocado.

Allergy Alert:

- No major allergens. Suitable for most dietary needs.

Substitutions for Vegans: Replace the chicken with mashed chickpeas mixed with vegan mayonnaise for a plant-based alternative.

Substitutions for Gluten Intolerance: No substitutions are needed; the recipe is gluten-free.

Vegetable Soup with Quinoa

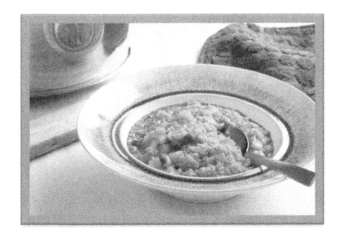

Recipe Description

Vegetable Soup with Quinoa is a light yet nourishing lunch option, ideal for seniors. This soup is packed with various vegetables and the added goodness of quinoa, making it a wholesome and diabetic-friendly meal.

Preparation Time: 15 min

Cooking Time: 30 min

Servings: 4

Glycemic Index: Low

Ingredients:

- 1/2 cup quinoa, rinsed
- 1 carrot, diced
- 1 celery stalk, diced
- 1 small onion, diced
- 1 zucchini, diced
- 2 tomatoes, diced
- 4 cups vegetable broth
- 1 tsp olive oil
- 1/2 tsp garlic powder
- 1/2 tsp dried basil
- Salt and pepper to taste

Directions

1. **Sauté Vegetables:** Heat the olive oil in a large pot over medium heat. Add the diced carrots, celery, and onion to the pot. Cook these **Ingredients:** for about 5 minutes, stirring occasionally, until they soften.
2. **Season the Vegetables:** Once the vegetables are slightly softened, stir in the garlic powder, dried basil, and a pinch of salt and pepper. Mix well to coat the vegetables with the seasonings evenly.
3. **Add Remaining Vegetables:** Add the diced zucchini and tomatoes to the pot. Stir to combine them with the other vegetables.
4. **Pour in the Broth:** Add the vegetable broth to the pot. Increase the heat to bring the mixture to a boil.
5. **Add Quinoa:** Once the soup is boiling, add the rinsed quinoa. Stir to distribute the quinoa evenly throughout the soup.
6. **Simmer the Soup:** Reduce the heat to a simmer. Let the soup cook for about 20 minutes or until the quinoa is fully cooked and the vegetables are tender.
7. **Serve:** Check the seasoning and adjust if necessary. The soup is ready to be served once the quinoa is cooked and the vegetables are tender. Serve it hot.

Nutritional Values (per serving)

Calories: 160, Protein: 6g, Carbohydrates: 28g, Fat: 3g, Fiber: 4g, Sodium: 480mg

Macronutrient Breakdown

Protein: 15%, Carbohydrates: 70%, Fat: 15%

Recipe Tips:

- Incorporate a variety of vegetables for a more diverse nutrient profile.
- Including quinoa adds protein and enhances the texture, making the soup more satisfying.

Allergy Alert:

- No major allergens. Suitable for most dietary needs.

Substitutions for Vegans: No substitutions are needed; the recipe is already vegan.

Substitutions for Gluten Intolerance: No substitutions are needed; the recipe is gluten-free.

Grilled Chicken Salad with Mixed Greens

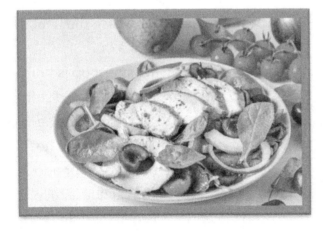

Recipe Description

This Grilled Chicken Salad with Mixed Greens is a perfect lunch for seniors seeking a light yet satisfying meal. The dish combines lean grilled chicken with a medley of fresh greens, offering a balanced, nutritious, diabetic-friendly option.

Preparation Time: 15 min

Cooking Time: 10 min (for grilling chicken)

Servings: 4

Glycemic Index: Low

Ingredients:

- 2 boneless, skinless chicken breasts
- 6 cups mixed greens (lettuce, spinach, arugula)
- 1 cucumber, sliced
- 1/2 red bell pepper, sliced
- 1/4 red onion, thinly sliced
- 2 tablespoons olive oil
- 1 tablespoon balsamic vinegar
- Salt and pepper to taste
- 1 teaspoon dried Italian herbs

Directions

1. **Season the Chicken:** Season the chicken breasts with salt, pepper, and dried Italian herbs. Ensure the chicken is evenly coated with the seasonings.
2. **Grill the Chicken:** Preheat the grill to medium heat. Place the seasoned chicken breasts on the grill. Cook them for about 5 minutes per side or until fully cooked through. The chicken should reach an internal temperature of 165°F (75°C).
3. **Rest and Slice the Chicken:** Once the chicken is grilled, transfer it to a cutting board and let it rest for a few minutes. Resting helps to keep the chicken juicy. After resting, slice the chicken into strips or bite-sized pieces.
4. **Prepare the Salad:** In a large salad bowl, combine the mixed greens, sliced

cucumber, sliced red bell pepper, and thinly sliced red onion.

5. **Make the Dressing:** Whisk together the olive oil and balsamic vinegar in a small bowl. This will be your salad dressing.

6. **Dress the Salad:** Drizzle the dressing over the mixed greens and vegetables. Toss the salad gently to ensure it's evenly coated with the dressing.

7. **Assemble the Salad:** Add the sliced grilled chicken to the salad.

8. **Serve:** Serve the salad immediately while the chicken is still warm and the greens are crisp.

Nutritional Values (per serving)

Calories: 200, Protein: 20g, Carbohydrates: 8g, Fat: 10g, Fiber: 2g, Sodium: 200mg

Macronutrient Breakdown

Protein: 40%, Carbohydrates: 16%, Fat: 44%

Recipe Tips:

- Allowing the chicken to rest after grilling ensures it remains juicy and flavorful.
- Add other vegetables, nuts, or seeds to the salad for texture, flavor, and nutrients.

Allergy Alert:

- No major allergens. Suitable for most dietary needs.

Substitutions for Vegans: Replace the chicken with grilled tofu or chickpeas for a plant-based protein source.

Substitutions for Gluten Intolerance: No substitutions are needed; the recipe is gluten-free.

Egg Salad on Whole Wheat Bread

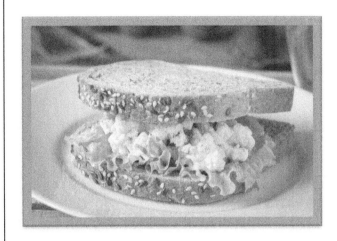

Recipe Description

Egg Salad on Whole Wheat Bread is a timeless American lunch, ideal for seniors. This simple yet delicious meal combines the protein-rich goodness of eggs with the fiber of whole wheat bread, creating a nutritious and diabetic-friendly option.

Preparation Time: 15 min

Cooking Time: 10 min (for boiling eggs)

Servings: 4

Glycemic Index: Low

Ingredients:

- 6 large eggs, hard-boiled and peeled
- 1/4 cup low-fat mayonnaise
- 1 tablespoon mustard
- 1/2 celery stalk, finely chopped
- Salt and pepper to taste
- 8 slices whole wheat bread
- Lettuce leaves and tomato slices (optional)

Directions

1. **Prepare the Eggs:** Place the eggs in a pot and cover them with cold water. Bring the water to a boil, then reduce the heat and simmer for 10 minutes. After boiling,

place the eggs in cold water to cool, then peel them.

2. **Chop the Eggs:** Chop the hard-boiled eggs into small pieces and transfer them to a mixing bowl.

3. **Make Egg Salad Mixture:** To the chopped eggs, add the low-fat mayonnaise, mustard, and finely chopped celery. Season the mixture with salt and pepper to taste. Mix well to combine all **Ingredients:** until the egg salad is creamy and evenly seasoned.

4. **Assemble the Sandwiches:** Lay out 4 slices of whole wheat bread. Spread the egg salad mixture evenly over these slices. Add lettuce leaves and tomato slices on top of the egg salad for extra freshness and flavor if desired.

5. **Complete the Sandwiches:** Top each sandwich with another slice of whole wheat bread. Press down gently to secure the fillings.

6. **Serve:** The sandwiches can be served immediately or wrapped and refrigerated until ready.

Nutritional Values (per serving)

Calories: 300, Protein: 20g, Carbohydrates: 28g, Fat: 12g, Fiber: 4g, Sodium: 400mg

Macronutrient Breakdown

Protein: 27%, Carbohydrates: 37%, Fat: 36%

Recipe Tips:

- Opt for low-fat mayonnaise to maintain a healthier profile.
- Adding mustard brings a tangy and flavorful touch to the egg salad.

Allergy Alert:

- Contains eggs and wheat. For a gluten-free option, substitute with gluten-free bread.

Substitutions for Vegans: Replace the egg salad with a tofu-based vegan egg salad alternative.

Substitutions for Gluten Intolerance: Use gluten-free bread.

Broccoli and Cheese Stuffed Baked Potatoes

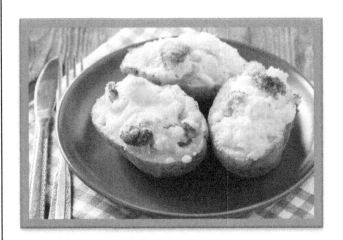

Recipe Description

Broccoli and cheese-stuffed baked potatoes are a comforting and nutritious lunch option for seniors. This dish combines the hearty flavor of baked potatoes with the health benefits of broccoli and the creamy goodness of cheese, making it both satisfying and diabetic-friendly.

Preparation Time: 10 min

Cooking Time: 45 min

Servings: 4

Glycemic Index: Low to Medium

Ingredients:

- 4 medium-sized russet potatoes
- 2 cups broccoli florets, steamed

- 1/2 cup low-fat cheddar cheese, shredded
- 1/4 cup low-fat milk
- 2 tablespoons unsalted butter
- Salt and pepper to taste

Directions

1. **Preheat the Oven:** Set your oven to 400°F (200°C). This high temperature is ideal for baking potatoes until they are soft and fluffy inside.
2. **Bake the Potatoes:** Clean the russet potatoes and pierce them several times with a fork. This allows steam to escape during baking. Place the potatoes on the oven rack and bake for about 45 minutes or until they are tender when pierced with a fork.
3. **Prepare the Potatoes:** Remove them from the oven once they are baked. Cut a slit along the top of each potato. Carefully scoop the insides into a bowl, leaving a thin layer of potato attached to the skin to maintain its structure.
4. **Make the Filling:** Mash the scooped potato in the bowl with low-fat milk, unsalted butter, salt, and pepper until smooth. Fold in the steamed broccoli florets and half of the shredded cheddar cheese.
5. **Stuff the Potatoes:** Spoon the broccoli and cheese potato mixture back into the skins. Distribute the filling evenly among the four potato skins.
6. **Add Cheese and Bake:** Sprinkle the remaining cheddar cheese on top of the stuffed potatoes. Please return them to the oven and bake for 10 minutes or until the cheese is melted and bubbly.
7. **Serve:** Remove them from the oven once the cheese is melted and the potatoes are heated through. Serve the stuffed potatoes hot.

Nutritional Values (per serving)

Calories: 250, Protein: 10g, Carbohydrates: 38g, Fat: 8g, Fiber: 5g, Sodium: 180mg

Macronutrient Breakdown

Protein: 16%, Carbohydrates: 61%, Fat: 23%

Recipe Tips:

- Baking the potatoes until they are soft ensures they are fluffy and easy to scoop.
- Steaming the broccoli helps to retain its nutrients and vibrant color.

Allergy Alert:

- Contains dairy. For a dairy-free version, use plant-based cheese and butter.

Substitutions for Vegans: Replace dairy cheese and butter with plant-based alternatives.

Substitutions for Gluten Intolerance: No substitutions are needed; the recipe is gluten-free.

Turkey and Cranberry Sandwich

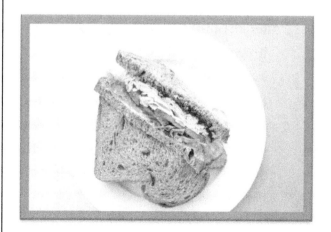

Recipe Description

The Turkey and Cranberry Sandwich is a classic American lunch, especially popular around the holidays but delightful any time of the year. It's a great choice for seniors, offering a good balance of protein from the turkey and a touch of sweetness from the cranberry.

Preparation Time: 10 min

Cooking Time: 0 min

Servings: 4

Glycemic Index: Low to Medium

Ingredients:

- 8 slices of whole wheat bread
- 8 ounces sliced turkey breast
- 1/4 cup cranberry sauce
- Lettuce leaves
- 2 tablespoons mayonnaise (optional)
- Salt and pepper to taste

Directions

1. **Prepare the Bread:** If you're using mayonnaise, spread a thin layer on one side of 4 slices of whole wheat bread. This adds flavor and moisture to the sandwich.

2. **Layer the Turkey:** Place the sliced turkey breast evenly on the 4 slices of bread with mayonnaise. The amount of turkey can be adjusted based on your preference.

3. **Add Cranberry Sauce:** Spoon a tablespoon of cranberry sauce over the turkey on each slice of bread. The cranberry sauce adds a sweet and tart flavor that complements the turkey.

4. **Include Lettuce:** Place lettuce leaves on top of the cranberry sauce. The lettuce adds freshness and a crunchy texture to the sandwich.

5. **Season:** Lightly season the filling with salt and pepper. This enhances the flavors of the turkey and cranberry.

6. **Complete the Sandwich:** Top each prepared slice of bread with another slice, forming 4 sandwiches in total.

7. **Cut and Serve:** Cut each sandwich in half diagonally or straight down the middle. Serve the sandwiches immediately for the best taste and texture.

Nutritional Values (per serving)

Calories: 250, Protein: 20g, Carbohydrates: 35g, Fat: 5g, Fiber: 5g, Sodium: 450mg

Macronutrient Breakdown

Protein: 32%, Carbohydrates: 56%, Fat: 12%

Recipe Tips:

- Choose low-sodium turkey breast to lower the overall sodium content of the sandwich.
- Opting for whole wheat bread adds a hearty flavor and increases the fiber content, which is beneficial for digestion.

Allergy Alert:

- Contains wheat. For a gluten-free option, substitute with gluten-free bread.

Substitutions for Vegans: Replace the turkey with a plant-based substitute, such as sliced tofu or a vegan deli slice, and use cranberry sauce that doesn't contain gelatin.

Substitutions for Gluten Intolerance: Use gluten free bread.

Spinach and Feta Cheese Wrap

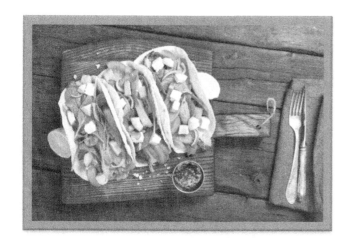

Recipe Description

The Spinach and Feta Cheese Wrap is a nutritious lunch for seniors. It combines the fresh taste of spinach with the tangy flavor of feta cheese, wrapped in a whole wheat tortilla for a satisfying and diabetic-friendly meal.

Preparation Time: 10 min

Cooking Time: 0 min

Servings: 4

Glycemic Index: Low

Ingredients:

- 4 whole wheat tortillas
- 2 cups fresh spinach leaves
- 1/2 cup feta cheese, crumbled
- 1/4 cup red onion, thinly sliced
- 1/4 cup cucumber, thinly sliced
- 2 tablespoons low-fat Greek yogurt
- 1 tablespoon olive oil
- Salt and pepper to taste

Directions

1. **Prepare the Tortillas:** Lay the whole wheat on a clean, flat surface. If the tortillas are stiff, warm them slightly in the microwave or on a skillet to make them more pliable.
2. **Add Greek Yogurt:** Spread a thin layer of low-fat Greek yogurt on each tortilla. This yogurt layer helps to bind the other **Ingredients:** and adds creaminess to the wrap.
3. **Layer the Ingredients::** Start by placing a layer of fresh spinach leaves on each tortilla. Then, add crumbled feta cheese, thinly sliced red onions, and cucumber slices over the spinach. Arrange these **Ingredients:** evenly to ensure each bite contains all the flavors.
4. **Season the Wrap:** Drizzle a bit of olive oil over the **Ingredients:** on each tortilla. Season with salt and pepper to enhance the flavors.
5. **Roll the Wraps:** Carefully roll up the tortillas tightly, tucking in the sides as you roll to secure the filling inside.
6. **Cut and Serve:** Once rolled, cut each wrap in half crosswise. This makes the wraps easier to handle and eat.
7. **Serve:** Serve the wraps immediately or in foil or plastic for a portable lunch option.

Nutritional Values (per serving)

Calories: 220, Protein: 8g, Carbohydrates: 28g, Fat: 9g, Fiber: 4g, Sodium: 400mg

Macronutrient Breakdown

Protein: 15%, Carbohydrates: 51%, Fat: 34%

Recipe Tips:

- Allowing the tortillas to reach room temperature before rolling helps prevent cracking.
- The Greek yogurt adds a creamy texture and can be enhanced with herbs or spices for additional flavor.

Allergy Alert:

- Contains wheat and dairy. For a dairy-free version, omit the feta cheese or use a dairy-free alternative.

Substitutions for Vegans: Replace feta cheese with vegan cheese and use a plant-based yogurt.

Substitutions for Gluten Intolerance: Use gluten-free tortillas.

Roasted Vegetable Quiche

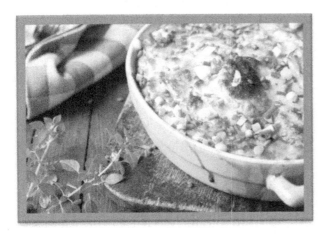

Recipe Description

The Roasted Vegetable Quiche is a delightful and nutritious lunch suitable for seniors. This dish features a medley of roasted vegetables in a light egg custard encased in a whole wheat crust, offering a balanced, hearty, and diabetic-friendly meal.

Preparation Time: 20 min

Cooking Time: 35 min

Servings: 4

Glycemic Index: Low to Medium

Ingredients:

- 1 premade whole wheat pie crust
- 1 cup mixed vegetables (bell peppers, zucchini, tomatoes), chopped
- 4 large eggs
- 1 cup low-fat milk
- 1/2 cup low-fat cheese, shredded
- 1 tablespoon olive oil
- Salt and pepper to taste
- 1/2 teaspoon dried herbs (such as thyme or oregano)

Directions

1. **Preheat the Oven:** Preheat your oven to 375°F (190°C). This temperature is optimal for baking the quiche.

2. **Prepare the Vegetables:** In a bowl, toss the chopped bell peppers, zucchini, and tomatoes with olive oil, salt, pepper, and dried herbs. Ensure the vegetables are evenly coated.

3. **Roast the Vegetables:** Spread the seasoned vegetables on a baking sheet. Roast them in the oven for 15 minutes until they are slightly tender. Remove the vegetables from the oven and set them aside.

4. **Prepare the Egg Mixture:** Whisk together the eggs and low-fat milk in a separate bowl. Season this mixture with salt and pepper to taste.

5. **Assemble the Quiche:** Place the premade whole wheat pie crust on a baking dish. Spread the roasted vegetables evenly in the pie crust.

6. **Add the Egg Mixture:** Pour the egg and milk mixture over the roasted vegetables in the pie crust. Make sure the mixture is evenly distributed.

7. **Add Cheese:** Sprinkle the shredded low-fat cheese over the quiche.

8. **Bake the Quiche:** Place the quiche in the oven and bake for 35 minutes, or until the custard is set and the top is lightly browned.

9. **Cool and Serve:** Allow the quiche to cool for a few minutes after baking. This makes it easier to slice and serve.

Nutritional Values (per serving)

Calories: 300, Protein: 12g, Carbohydrates: 25g, Fat: 18g, Fiber: 3g, Sodium: 350mg

Macronutrient Breakdown

Protein: 16%, Carbohydrates: 33%, Fat: 51%

Recipe Tips:

- You can vary the vegetables according to the season or your preference.
- Allowing the quiche to cool slightly after baking will make it easier to slice and serve without falling apart.

Allergy Alert:

- Contains wheat, eggs, and dairy. For a dairy-free version, use plant-based milk and cheese.

Substitutions for Vegans: Use a vegan egg substitute and plant-based milk and cheese. Substitutions for Gluten Intolerance: Use a gluten-free pie crust.

Black Bean and Corn Salad

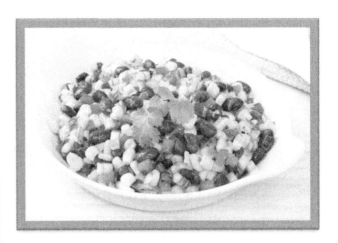

Recipe Description

The Black Bean and Corn Salad is a vibrant and flavorful lunch option, ideal for seniors. This salad is full of fiber and protein from black beans, and the sweetness of corn provides a delightful contrast. It's a nutritious, light, and diabetic-friendly meal.

Preparation Time: 15 min

Cooking Time: 0 min

Servings: 4

Glycemic Index: Low

Ingredients:

- 1 can black beans, rinsed and drained
- 1 cup corn kernels, fresh or frozen (thawed if frozen)
- 1 red bell pepper, diced
- 1/2 red onion, finely chopped
- 1/4 cup cilantro, chopped
- 2 tablespoons lime juice
- 1 tablespoon olive oil
- 1/2 teaspoon cumin
- Salt and pepper to taste

Directions

1. **Combine Salad Ingredients::** In a large bowl, mix the rinsed and drained black beans, corn kernels, diced red bell pepper, and finely chopped red onion.

2. **Prepare the Dressing:** In a separate small bowl, whisk together lime juice, olive oil, and cumin. Add salt and pepper to taste. This dressing will bring a bright and tangy flavor to the salad.

3. **Dress the Salad:** Pour the prepared dressing over the black bean and corn mixture in the large bowl. Toss the salad gently to ensure all **Ingredients:** are evenly coated with the dressing.

4. **Add Cilantro:** Stir in the chopped cilantro to add a fresh and herby flavor to the salad.

5. **Chill the Salad:** Refrigerate the salad for at least 30 minutes. This chilling time allows the flavors to meld together beautifully.

6. **Serving:** Serve the salad chilled or at room temperature, depending on your preference.

Nutritional Values (per serving)

Calories: 180, Protein: 8g, Carbohydrates: 30g, Fat: 5g, Fiber: 8g, Sodium: 200mg

Macronutrient Breakdown

Protein: 18%, Carbohydrates: 67%, Fat: 15%

Recipe Tips:

- Opt for fresh corn kernels in season for a sweeter and more vibrant flavor.
- The salad can be prepared and stored in the refrigerator, making it convenient for up to two days.

Allergy Alert:

- No major allergens. Suitable for most dietary needs.

Substitutions for Vegans: No substitutions are needed; the recipe is already vegan-friendly.

Substitutions for Gluten Intolerance: No substitutions are needed; the recipe is gluten-free.

CHAPTER 4: DELICIOUS AND HEALTHY DINNERS

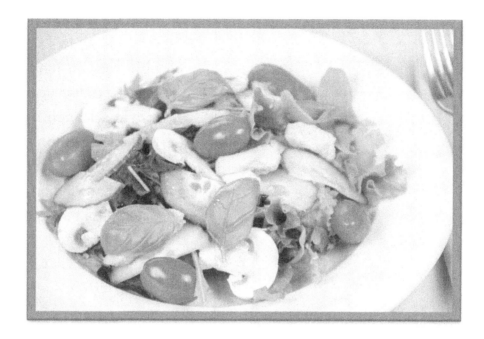

Good food is beneficial for several reasons, including weight loss, more energy, and keeping fit. You don't even need a reason to prepare these wholesome meal suggestions. You may feel good about what you're serving for supper if you only add a couple of them to your weeknight rotation.

Ensure that the healthy supper suggestions you'll discover here are as fulfilling as the decadent meals you're already familiar with and enjoy; they've been slightly adjusted so that you and your family get the nutrition they need for the upcoming week.

These recipes (ranging from simple fish dishes to slow cooker chicken recipes, grain bowls, and spinach salads) all share guilt-free deliciousness.

Baked Lemon Garlic Tilapia

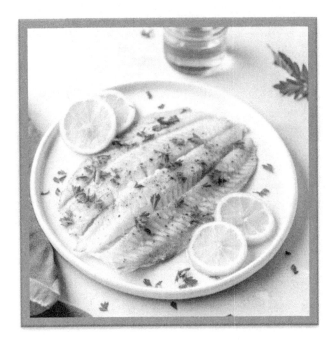

Recipe Description

Baked Lemon Garlic Tilapia is a light and flavorful dinner option for seniors. This dish features the delicate taste of tilapia enhanced with the zest of lemon and the warmth of garlic, making it a healthy and diabetic-friendly choice.

Preparation Time: 10 min

Cooking Time: 20 min

Servings: 4

Glycemic Index: Low

Ingredients:

- 4 tilapia fillets
- 2 lemons, one juiced and one sliced
- 3 cloves garlic, minced
- 2 tablespoons olive oil
- 1 tablespoon fresh parsley, chopped
- Salt and pepper to taste

Directions

1. **Preheat the Oven:** Preheat your oven to 400°F (200°C). This temperature is ideal for baking the fish to perfection without drying it out.
2. **Prepare the Baking Dish:** Place the tilapia fillets in a single layer in a baking dish. You can lightly grease the dish with olive oil or line it with parchment paper for easy cleanup.
3. **Make the Lemon Garlic Mixture:** In a small bowl, whisk together olive oil, the juice of one lemon, minced garlic, and a pinch of salt and pepper. This mixture will be used to flavor the tilapia.
4. **Season the Tilapia:** Pour the lemon garlic mixture evenly over the tilapia fillets, ensuring each fillet is well-coated. This will infuse the fish with a bright, tangy flavor.
5. **Add Lemon Slices:** Thinly slice the remaining lemon and arrange the slices on top of the seasoned fillets. The lemon slices add additional lemon flavor and make for an attractive presentation.
6. **Bake the Tilapia:** Place the baking dish in the preheated oven. Bake the tilapia for approximately 20 minutes. The fish is done when it flakes easily with a fork and is opaque throughout.
7. **Garnish and Serve:** Remove the dish from the oven once the tilapia is cooked. Sprinkle the freshly chopped parsley over the fillets for garnish, adding color and freshness.
8. **Serving Suggestions:** Serve the baked lemon garlic tilapia hot, perhaps with steamed vegetables or a light salad for a complete meal.

Nutritional Values (per serving)

Calories: 180, Protein: 23g, Carbohydrates: 2g, Fat: 9g, Fiber: 0g, Sodium: 60mg

Macronutrient Breakdown

Protein: 51%, Carbohydrates: 4%, Fat: 45%

Recipe Tips:

- Using fresh tilapia ensures the best flavor and texture.
- The lemon juice not only adds freshness but also helps balance the fish's richness.

Allergy Alert:

- Contains fish. Suitable for most other dietary needs.

Substitutions for Vegans: Replace tilapia with a firm tofu or a vegan fish alternative.

Substitutions for Gluten Intolerance: No substitutions are needed; the recipe is gluten-free.

Grilled Chicken and Vegetable Skewers

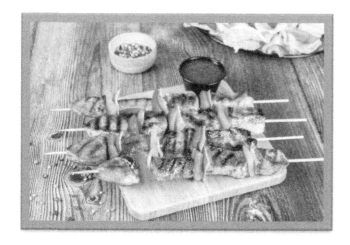

Recipe Description

Grilled Chicken and Vegetable Skewers are a delightful dinner option for seniors, offering a perfect balance of lean protein and fresh vegetables. This meal is nutritious and adds a fun and interactive element to dining, making it a great choice for a healthy and diabetic-friendly dinner.

Preparation Time: 20 min (plus marinating time)

Cooking Time: 10 min

Servings: 4

Glycemic Index: Low

Ingredients:

- 2 boneless, skinless chicken breasts cut into cubes
- 1 zucchini, sliced
- 1 bell pepper, cut into pieces
- 1 red onion, cut into wedges
- 1/4 cup olive oil
- 2 tablespoons lemon juice
- 1 teaspoon dried oregano
- 1 garlic clove, minced
- Salt and pepper to taste
- Wooden or metal skewers

Directions

1. **Marinate the Chicken:** In a mixing bowl, whisk together olive oil, lemon juice, dried oregano, minced garlic, and a pinch of salt and pepper. Add the cubed chicken breasts to the bowl, ensuring they are fully coated with the marinade. Cover and refrigerate for at least 30 minutes. Marinating the chicken will infuse it with flavor and tenderize it.

2. **Prepare the Vegetables:** While the chicken is marinating, prepare the vegetables. Wash and slice the zucchini, cut the bell pepper into uniform pieces, and cut the red onion into wedges. The

vegetables should be roughly the same size for even cooking.

3. **Preheat the Grill:** Preheat your grill to medium-high heat. This temperature is ideal for cooking the skewers evenly without burning them.

4. **Assemble the Skewers:** If using wooden skewers, soak them in water for at least 20 minutes before grilling to prevent them from burning. Thread the marinated chicken, zucchini slices, bell pepper pieces, and red onion wedges onto the skewers, alternating between the chicken and vegetables.

5. **Grill the Skewers:** Place the skewers on the grill. Grill them for about 10 minutes, turning occasionally, until the chicken is thoroughly cooked and the vegetables are tender. The chicken should reach an internal temperature of 165°F (75°C).

6. **Serve:** Once cooked, remove the skewers from the grill. Let them rest for a couple of minutes before serving.

Nutritional Values (per serving)
Calories: 250, Protein: 22g, Carbohydrates: 6g, Fat: 15g, Fiber: 2g, Sodium: 70mg
Macronutrient Breakdown
Protein: 35%, Carbohydrates: 10%, Fat: 55%

Recipe Tips:
- Marinating the chicken adds flavor and tenderness. Marinate for at least 30 minutes or up to several hours for best results.
- Use a variety of vegetables for a colorful and nutrient-rich meal. You can add or substitute other vegetables like mushrooms or cherry tomatoes.

Allergy Alert:
- No major allergens. Suitable for most dietary needs.

Substitutions for Vegans: Replace chicken with tofu or a variety of vegetables.

Substitutions for Gluten Intolerance: No substitutions are needed; the recipe is gluten-free.

Turkey Meatloaf with Sweet Potato Topping

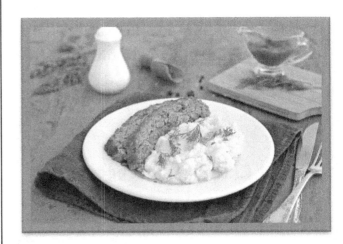

Recipe Description
Turkey Meatloaf with Sweet Potato Topping is a hearty and nutritious dinner for seniors. This twist on a traditional meatloaf uses lean turkey meat and is topped with a sweet potato mash, offering a balanced and diabetic-friendly meal.

Preparation Time: 20 min
Cooking Time: 45 min
Servings: 4
Glycemic Index: Low to Medium

Ingredients:
- 1 lb ground turkey
- 1 sweet potato, peeled and cubed

- 1 onion, finely chopped
- 1 carrot, grated
- 1 celery stalk, finely chopped
- 2 cloves garlic, minced
- 1 egg, beaten
- 1/4 cup whole wheat breadcrumbs
- 1/4 cup low-fat milk
- 1 tablespoon olive oil
- 1 teaspoon dried thyme
- Salt and pepper to taste

Directions

1. **Preheat** the oven to 375°F (190°C).
2. **Boil** sweet potato cubes until tender, then mash.
3. **Sauté** onion, carrot, celery, and garlic in olive oil until softened.
4. **Combine** ground turkey, sautéed vegetables, egg, breadcrumbs, milk, thyme, salt, and pepper in a bowl.
5. **Press** the turkey mixture into a loaf pan.
6. **Spread** the mashed sweet potato on top of the meatloaf.
7. **Bake** for 45 minutes or until the meatloaf is cooked through.
8. **Let cool** for a few minutes before slicing and serving.

Nutritional Values (per serving)

Calories: 280, Protein: 24g, Carbohydrates: 20g, Fat: 12g, Fiber: 3g, Sodium: 200mg
Macronutrient Breakdown
Protein: 34%, Carbohydrates: 29%, Fat: 37%

Recipe Tips:

- Using sweet potatoes instead of regular potatoes adds a natural sweetness and more nutrients.

- Ensure the meatloaf is fully cooked by checking the internal temperature, which reaches 165°F (75°C).

Allergy Alert:

- Contains wheat and eggs. For a gluten-free option, use gluten-free breadcrumbs.

Substitutions for Vegans: Replace ground turkey with a mixture of lentils and quinoa, and use a flax egg.
Substitutions for Gluten Intolerance: Use gluten-free breadcrumbs.

Baked Salmon with Roasted Asparagus

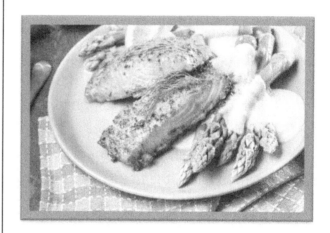

Recipe Description

Baked Salmon with Roasted Asparagus is a simple yet elegant dinner for seniors. This dish combines omega-3-rich salmon with nutrient-packed asparagus, creating a meal that is not only delicious but also beneficial for a diabetic-friendly diet.

Preparation Time: 10 min
Cooking Time: 20 min
Servings: 4
Glycemic Index: Low
Ingredients:

- 4 salmon fillets
- 1 bunch of asparagus, trimmed
- 2 tablespoons olive oil
- 1 lemon, half juiced and half sliced
- 2 cloves garlic, minced
- Salt and pepper to taste
- Fresh dill for garnish (optional)

Directions

1. **Preheat the Oven:** Start by setting your oven to 400°F (200°C). This temperature is ideal for baking the salmon while roasting the asparagus perfectly.

2. **Prepare the Baking Sheet:** Line a baking sheet with parchment paper for easy cleanup. Place the salmon fillets on the sheet, ensuring they have enough space between them for even cooking.

3. **Season the Salmon:** Mix half the olive oil with the juice of half a lemon in a small bowl. Add the minced garlic to this mixture. Brush this mixture over the salmon fillets, then season them with salt and pepper to taste.

4. **Prepare the Asparagus:** Trim the ends and place them in a bowl. Toss them with the remaining olive oil, ensuring they are lightly coated. Arrange the asparagus around the salmon fillets on the baking sheet.

5. **Add Lemon Slices:** Thinly slice the remaining half of the lemon and place the slices on top of the salmon fillets. This adds a fresh, zesty flavor as the salmon bakes.

6. **Bake the Dish:** Place the baking sheet in the preheated oven. Bake for about 20 minutes. The salmon should be cooked through and flaked easily with a fork, and the asparagus should be tender yet crisp.

7. **Garnishing:** Once cooked, remove the baking sheet from the oven. If desired, garnish the salmon with fresh dill for an added touch of flavor and presentation.

8. **Serve:** Serve the baked salmon and roasted asparagus hot, ideally immediately after cooking, for the best taste and texture.

Nutritional Values (per serving)

Calories: 300, Protein: 25g, Carbohydrates: 6g, Fat: 20g, Fiber: 2g, Sodium: 70mg

Macronutrient Breakdown

Protein: 33%, Carbohydrates: 8%, Fat: 59%

Recipe Tips:

- The lemon juice adds a fresh zest to the salmon.
- Be careful not to overcook the salmon to maintain its tenderness and moisture.

Allergy Alert:

- Contains fish. Suitable for most other dietary needs.

Substitutions for Vegans: Replace salmon with a large portobello mushroom cap or tofu slices.

Substitutions for Gluten Intolerance: No substitutions are needed; the recipe is gluten-free.

Vegetarian Stuffed Peppers

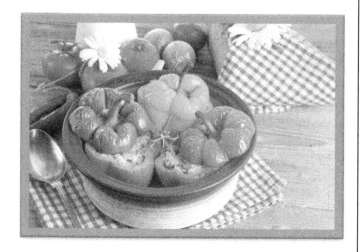

Recipe Description

Vegetarian Stuffed Peppers are a colorful and hearty dinner option for seniors. These peppers are filled with a savory mix of vegetables, rice, and beans, providing a nutrient-rich meal that is both diabetic-friendly and satisfying.

Preparation Time: 20 min

Cooking Time: 30 min

Servings: 4

Glycemic Index: Low

Ingredients:

- 4 bell peppers, tops removed and seeded
- 1 cup cooked brown rice
- 1 can black beans, rinsed and drained
- 1 cup corn kernels, fresh or frozen
- 1/2 cup onion, chopped
- 1/2 cup tomato, diced
- 1 teaspoon cumin
- 1 teaspoon paprika
- 1/2 cup low-fat shredded cheese
- Salt and pepper to taste
- 2 tablespoons olive oil

Directions

1. **Preheat the Oven:** Begin by heating your oven to 375°F (190°C). This temperature allows the peppers to cook thoroughly without burning.
2. **Prepare the Filling:** In a large mixing bowl, combine the cooked brown rice, black beans, corn kernels, chopped onion, and diced tomato. Add cumin, paprika, and a pinch of salt and pepper to taste. Mix these **Ingredients:** well to ensure the flavors are evenly distributed.
3. **Prepare the Bell Peppers:** Wash them and cut off their tops. Remove the seeds and any membranes from inside the peppers. Lightly drizzle the inside of each pepper with olive oil. This helps to keep them moist while baking.
4. **Stuff the Peppers:** Spoon the rice and bean mixture into each bell pepper, packing it down gently until it's just below the top of each pepper.
5. **Bake the Peppers:** Place the stuffed peppers upright in a baking dish. Cover the dish with aluminum foil to prevent excessive browning or drying out.
6. **Baking Time:** Bake the peppers in the preheated oven for 25 minutes. The covering helps steam the peppers, making them tender.
7. **Add Cheese:** After 25 minutes, remove the foil and sprinkle each pepper with shredded cheese. Return the baking dish to the oven, uncovered, and bake for 5 minutes or until the cheese is melted and bubbly.
8. **Serving:** Remove the peppers from the oven once the cheese is melted. Let them

cool for a few minutes before serving, as they will be hot.

Nutritional Values (per serving)

Calories: 260, Protein: 10g, Carbohydrates: 38g, Fat: 9g, Fiber: 8g, Sodium: 300mg

Macronutrient Breakdown

Protein: 15%, Carbohydrates: 58%, Fat: 27%

Recipe Tips:

- Choose bell peppers of various colors for a visually appealing dish.
- The filling can be customized with different vegetables or spices according to preference.

Allergy Alert:

- Contains dairy. For a dairy-free version, use a dairy-free cheese alternative.

Substitutions for Vegans: Use vegan cheese instead of low-fat cheese.

Substitutions for Gluten Intolerance: No substitutions are needed; the recipe is gluten-free.

Shrimp and Broccoli Stir-Fry

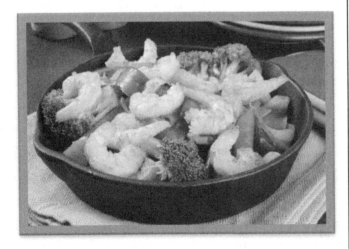

Recipe Description

Shrimp and Broccoli Stir-Fry is a quick and delicious dinner choice for seniors. This dish features tender shrimp, and nutrient-rich broccoli stir-fried in a savory sauce, making it a healthy and diabetic-friendly option.

Preparation Time: 15 min

Cooking Time: 10 min

Servings: 4

Glycemic Index: Low

Ingredients:

- 1 lb shrimp, peeled and deveined
- 2 cups broccoli florets
- 1 red bell pepper, sliced
- 1 garlic clove, minced
- 2 tablespoons soy sauce (low sodium)
- 1 tablespoon sesame oil
- 1 teaspoon ginger, grated
- 1 tablespoon olive oil
- Salt and pepper to taste

Directions

1. **Prepare Ingredients::** Start by preparing your **Ingredients:**. Peel and devein the shrimp if not already done. Wash and cut the broccoli into florets, slice the red bell pepper into thin strips, mince the garlic, and grate the ginger.
2. **Heat the Skillet:** Place a large skillet or wok over medium-high heat. Add olive oil to the pan, swirling to coat the surface.
3. **Stir-Fry Garlic and Ginger:** Add minced garlic and grated ginger to the skillet. Stir-fry for about 30 seconds. Be careful not to burn the garlic.
4. **Cook the Shrimp:** Add the shrimp to the skillet. Cook for 2-3 minutes, stirring frequently, until the shrimp turn pink and

are cooked through. Avoid overcooking to keep the shrimp tender.

5. **Remove Shrimp:** Once cooked, remove them from the skillet and set them aside on a plate. This prevents them from overcooking while you cook the vegetables.

6. **Stir-Fry Vegetables:** Add broccoli florets and sliced red bell pepper in the same skillet. Stir-fry for about 5 minutes or until the vegetables are tender but crisp.

7. **Combine Shrimp and Vegetables:** Return the cooked shrimp to the skillet with the vegetables.

8. **Add Sauce:** Pour the low-sodium soy sauce and sesame oil over the shrimp and vegetables. Toss everything to combine and ensure the **Ingredients:** are evenly coated with the sauce.

9. **Season:** Season the stir-fry with salt and pepper to taste. Adjust seasoning according to your preference.

10. **Serve:** Remove the skillet from heat once everything is heated through and well mixed. Serve the shrimp and broccoli stir-fry hot.

Nutritional Values (per serving)

Calories: 220, Protein: 24g, Carbohydrates: 8g, Fat: 10g, Fiber: 2g, Sodium: 350mg

Macronutrient Breakdown

Protein: 44%, Carbohydrates: 15%, Fat: 41%

Recipe Tips:

- Cook shrimp until just pink to avoid overcooking, as overcooked shrimp can become rubbery.
- The addition of ginger adds a fresh and zesty flavor to the dish.

Allergy Alert:

- Contains shellfish and soy. For a soy-free version, use coconut aminos.

Substitutions for Vegans: Replace shrimp with tofu or a vegan shrimp alternative.

Substitutions for Gluten Intolerance: Use gluten-free soy sauce.

Beef and Vegetable Stew

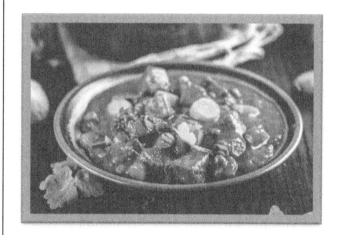

Recipe Description

Beef and Vegetable Stew is a classic and comforting dinner for seniors. This hearty stew combines tender beef with various vegetables in a rich broth, providing a warm and satisfying meal that's both nutritious and diabetic-friendly.

Preparation Time: 20 min

Cooking Time: 2 hours

Servings: 4

Glycemic Index: Low

Ingredients:

- 1 lb beef stew meat, cut into cubes
- 2 carrots, peeled and sliced
- 2 potatoes, peeled and diced
- 1 onion, chopped
- 2 celery stalks, sliced

- 4 cups beef broth
- 1 can diced tomatoes
- 1 teaspoon dried thyme
- 1 bay leaf
- 2 tablespoons olive oil
- Salt and pepper to taste

Directions

1. **Prepare the Ingredients::** Cut beef stew meat into uniform cubes. Peel and slice the carrots, peel and dice the potatoes, chop the onion, and slice the celery stalks.

2. **Brown the Beef:** Heat olive oil in a large pot over medium-high heat. Add the beef cubes to the pot and cook them until they're browned on all sides. This browning process adds flavor to the meat and the stew.

3. **Sauté the Aromatics:** Add the chopped onions to the pot once the beef is browned. Sauté until the onions are translucent and softened. If you're using garlic (as mentioned in the **Recipe Tips:** but not listed in the **Ingredients:**), add minced garlic at this stage and cook it with the onions until fragrant.

4. **Add Broth and Vegetables:** Pour the beef broth into the pot. Add the diced tomatoes (with their juice), sliced carrots, and diced potatoes and celery. Stir the mixture to combine the **Ingredients:**.

5. **Season the Stew:** Add the dried thyme and bay leaf to the pot. Season the stew with salt and pepper to taste. Stir well.

6. **Simmer the Stew:** Bring the stew to a boil. Once it reaches a boil, reduce the heat to low, cover the pot, and let the stew simmer. Allow it to cook for about 2 hours. Slow cooking helps the beef become tender, and the flavors meld together.

7. **Final Seasoning:** After 2 hours, check the stew for seasoning. Adjust the salt and pepper if needed.

8. **Remove Bay Leaf:** Remove the bay leaf from the stew before serving.

9. **Serve the Stew:** Serve the beef and vegetable stew hot. It's hearty enough to be a meal on its own.

Nutritional Values (per serving)

Calories: 320, Protein: 25g, Carbohydrates: 20g, Fat: 15g, Fiber: 3g, Sodium: 600mg

Macronutrient Breakdown

Protein: 31%, Carbohydrates: 25%, Fat: 44%

Recipe Tips:

- Slow cooking the stew allows the flavors to meld and the beef to become tender.
- This stew can be made in a slow cooker for convenience. If using a slow cooker, combine all **Ingredients:** in the slow cooker and cook on low for 6-8 hours or on high for 3-4 hours.

Allergy Alert:

- No major allergens. Suitable for most dietary needs.

Substitutions for Vegans: Replace beef with a plant-based meat alternative and use vegetable broth.

Substitutions for Gluten Intolerance: Ensure beef broth is gluten-free.

Baked Cod with Herb Crust

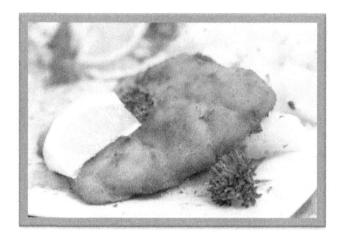

Recipe Description

Baked Cod with Herb Crust is a light, healthy dinner option for seniors. The dish features flaky cod topped with a flavorful herb crust, offering a tasty and diabetic-friendly meal that's easy to prepare.

Preparation Time: 15 min

Cooking Time: 20 min

Servings: 4

Glycemic Index: Low

Ingredients:

- 4 cod fillets
- 1/2 cup whole wheat breadcrumbs
- 2 tablespoons parsley, finely chopped
- 1 teaspoon lemon zest
- 1 garlic clove, minced
- 2 tablespoons olive oil
- Salt and pepper to taste

Directions

1. **Preheat the Oven:** Preheat your oven to 400°F (200°C). This temperature is ideal for baking the cod to perfection.
2. **Prepare the Herb Crust Mixture:** In a medium-sized bowl, combine the whole wheat breadcrumbs, finely chopped parsley, lemon zest, and minced garlic. Add a pinch of salt and pepper to this mixture. Mix these **Ingredients:** well until you have a uniform breadcrumb mixture. The lemon zest will add a fresh flavor to the crust.
3. **Prepare the Cod Fillets:** Brush each cod fillet lightly with olive oil. The olive oil adds flavor and helps the breadcrumb mixture stick to the fish.
4. **Apply the Herb Crust:** Press the breadcrumb mixture onto the top of each oiled cod fillet. Make sure to cover the surface evenly for a consistent crust.
5. **Bake the Cod:** Line a baking sheet with parchment paper and place the breadcrumb-coated cod fillets on it. The parchment paper prevents sticking and allows for easy cleanup. Bake the cod in the preheated oven for 20 minutes. The goal is to cook the fish until it flakes easily with a fork and the crust turns golden brown.
6. **Serving:** Once baked, remove the cod from the oven. Serve the fillets hot, and if desired, garnish with lemon wedges. The lemon wedges can be squeezed over the fish for extra zest.

Nutritional Values (per serving)

Calories: 200, Protein: 22g, Carbohydrates: 10g, Fat: 8g, Fiber: 1g, Sodium: 150mg

Macronutrient Breakdown

Protein: 44%, Carbohydrates: 20%, Fat: 36%

Recipe Tips:

- The lemon zest in the breadcrumb mixture adds a fresh and zesty flavor to the fish.
- Be careful not to overcook the cod to maintain its moisture and flakiness. Overcooked cod can become dry.

Allergy Alert:
- Contains fish and wheat. For a gluten-free option, use gluten-free breadcrumbs.

Substitutions for Vegans: Replace cod with thick tofu slices or a vegan fish alternative. Substitutions for Gluten Intolerance: Use gluten-free breadcrumbs.

Vegetarian Chili

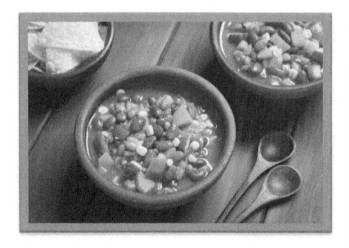

Recipe Description
Vegetarian Chili is a hearty and warming dinner, perfect for seniors. This dish is packed with various beans and vegetables, offering a high-fiber, nutritious, and diabetic-friendly meal that's both satisfying and flavorful.

Preparation Time: 20 min

Cooking Time: 1 hour

Servings: 4

Glycemic Index: Low

60

Ingredients:
- 1 can black beans, rinsed and drained
- 1 can kidney beans, rinsed and drained
- 1 can dice tomatoes
- 1 onion, chopped
- 1 bell pepper, chopped
- 2 cloves garlic, minced
- 2 carrots, diced
- 1 zucchini, diced
- 2 tablespoons tomato paste
- 1 tablespoon chili powder
- 1 teaspoon cumin
- 1 teaspoon paprika
- 2 cups vegetable broth
- Salt and pepper to taste
- 2 tablespoons olive oil

Directions
1. **Prepare the Vegetables:** Begin by chopping the onion, bell pepper, carrots, and zucchini into bite-sized pieces. Mince the garlic cloves finely.
2. **Sauté Aromatics:** Heat the olive oil over medium heat in a large pot. Add the chopped onions and minced garlic. Sauté them until the onions become translucent and fragrant, about 3-4 minutes.
3. **Add Vegetables:** To the pot, add the chopped bell peppers, carrots, and zucchini. Cook for another 5 minutes, stirring occasionally, until the vegetables soften.
4. **Mix in Beans and Tomatoes:** Drain and rinse the black and kidney beans. Add them to the pot along with the can of diced tomatoes (including the juice). Stir well to combine.

5. **Season the Chili:** Add the tomato paste, chili powder, cumin, and paprika to the pot. Mix thoroughly so that the spices are evenly distributed.
6. **Add Broth and Simmer:** Pour in the vegetable broth. Bring the mixture to a boil, then reduce the heat to low. Allow the chili to simmer uncovered for about 1 hour. Stir occasionally to prevent sticking and ensure even cooking.
7. **Seasoning and Serving:** After the chili has thickened and the vegetables are tender, taste and adjust the seasoning with salt and pepper. Serve the chili hot. For an added touch, you can top it with low-fat sour cream or shredded cheese if desired.

Nutritional Values (per serving)

Calories: 280, Protein: 14g, Carbohydrates: 45g, Fat: 7g, Fiber: 13g, Sodium: 500mg

Macronutrient Breakdown

Protein: 20%, Carbohydrates: 64%, Fat: 16%

Recipe Tips:
- Allowing the chili to simmer for an hour helps develop a rich flavor profile.
- This chili can be stored in the refrigerator for several days, and the flavors often improve the next day.

Allergy Alert:
- No major allergens. Suitable for most dietary needs.

Substitutions for Vegans: No substitutions are needed; the recipe is already vegan.

Substitutions for Gluten Intolerance: No substitutions are needed; the recipe is gluten-free.

Herb Roasted Chicken with Vegetables

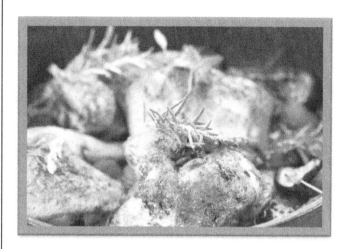

Recipe Description

Herb Roasted Chicken with Vegetables is a classic and comforting dinner choice for seniors. This one-pan meal combines succulent chicken with a medley of roasted vegetables, all seasoned with aromatic herbs, creating a nutritious and diabetic-friendly dish.

Preparation Time: 15 min

Cooking Time: 1 hour

Servings: 4

Glycemic Index: Low

Ingredients:
- 4 chicken thighs, bone-in and skin-on
- 2 carrots, peeled and sliced
- 2 potatoes, diced
- 1 onion, quartered
- 2 tablespoons olive oil
- 1 teaspoon dried rosemary
- 1 teaspoon dried thyme
- 1 garlic clove, minced
- Salt and pepper to taste

Directions

1. **Preheat Oven:** Preheat your oven to 375°F (190°C). This temperature is ideal for roasting both the chicken and vegetables evenly.
2. **Prepare the Vegetables:** Peel and slice the carrots, dice the potatoes, and quarter the onion. Placing the vegetables in a large bowl, toss them with one tablespoon of olive oil, half the amount of rosemary, half the thyme, half the minced garlic, and a pinch of salt and pepper. This ensures the vegetables are evenly coated with the seasoning.
3. **Arrange Vegetables in Roasting Pan:** Spread the seasoned vegetables in a single layer on a large roasting pan. This allows them to cook evenly and become tender.
4. **Season the Chicken:** In a separate bowl, season the chicken thighs with the remaining olive oil, rosemary, thyme, garlic, and a generous pinch of salt and pepper. Make sure the chicken is evenly coated with the herb mixture.
5. **Place Chicken on Vegetables:** Lay the seasoned chicken thighs skin-side up over the bed of vegetables in the roasting pan. Placing the chicken on top allows the juices to drip down and flavor the vegetables as they cook.
6. **Roast:** Place the roasting pan in the preheated oven. Roast for approximately 1 hour. The chicken should be cooked through (reaching an internal temperature of 165°F or 75°C), and the vegetables should be tender and caramelized.
7. **Serving:** Once cooked, remove the pan from the oven. Let it cool slightly for a few minutes, then serve hot directly from the pan.

Nutritional Values (per serving)

Calories: 350, Protein: 25g, Carbohydrates: 20g, Fat: 20g, Fiber: 3g, Sodium: 200mg

Macronutrient Breakdown

Protein: 29%, Carbohydrates: 23%, Fat: 48%

Recipe Tips:

- Roasting the chicken on top of the vegetables allows the juices to flavor them, enhancing their taste.
- The skin-on chicken thighs remain moist and flavorful during roasting, providing a delicious texture and taste.

Allergy Alert:

- No major allergens. Suitable for most dietary needs.

Substitutions for Vegans: Replace chicken with portobello mushrooms or a vegan meat substitute.

Substitutions for Gluten Intolerance: No substitutions are needed; the recipe is gluten-free.

CHAPTER 5: SNACKS AND TREATS

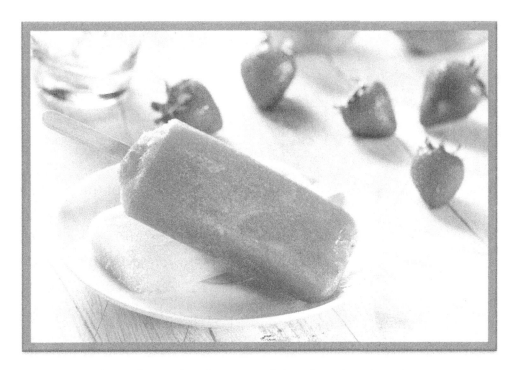

It's crucial to prioritize nutrient-dense foods most of the time, but it's also necessary to occasionally indulge in your favorite foods in moderation. Selecting a healthy sugar substitute when you crave will help you stick to your diet and nutrition plan. Fruit's naturally occurring sugars contain other health-promoting elements. However, added sugars—that is, sugars added to our food— additionally provide empty calories and no nutrition.

Over time, consuming excessive amounts of added sugar has been linked to increased incidences of hypertension, diabetes, and inflammation, among other health issues. Furthermore, the average American eats seventy-seven grams of sugar daily, more than three times the amount that the American Heart Association advises.

Nutrition experts recommend searching for sweet snacks with minimal added sugar and a ratio of protein to healthy fats to keep you satisfied and vigorous. But most importantly, it must be delectable; gladly, nutritious food can and should be tasty! I've compiled the top healthy sweet treats to satisfy any hunger, including "nice cream" and healthier fruit roll-ups.

Apple Cinnamon Yogurt Parfait

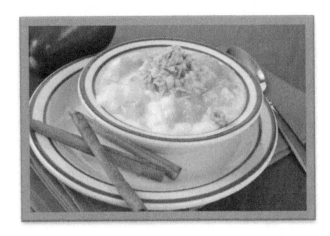

Recipe Description

Apple Cinnamon Yogurt Parfait is a delightful and nutritious snack or treat for seniors. It layers Greek yogurt with cinnamon-spiced apples and granola, offering a delicious combination of textures and flavors that's both healthy and diabetic-friendly.

Preparation Time: 10 min

Cooking Time: 0 min

Servings: 4

Glycemic Index: Low

Ingredients:

- 2 cups Greek yogurt, low-fat
- 2 apples, diced
- 1 teaspoon cinnamon
- 1 cup granola
- 1 tablespoon honey or sugar-free syrup (optional)

Directions

1. **Prepare the Apples:** Start by washing the apples thoroughly. Dice them into small, bite-sized pieces. Removing the skin is optional; keeping it on adds extra fiber.

2. **Spice the Apples:** Toss the diced apples with a teaspoon of cinnamon in a mixing bowl. Make sure the apple pieces are evenly coated with cinnamon. This not only adds flavor but also a pleasant aroma.

3. **Layer the Parfait:** Select serving glasses or bowls for the parfaits. Begin layering by spooning a portion of the Greek yogurt into each glass. Aim for about a quarter of the yogurt in each to start.

4. **Add Spiced Apples:** Add a layer of the cinnamon-spiced apples on top of the yogurt layer.

5. **Add Granola:** Follow the apple layer with a layer of granola. If you prefer a crunchier texture, add a generous amount of granola.

6. **Repeat Layers:** Repeat the layers of yogurt, spiced apples, and granola until the glasses are filled to the top. Depending on the size of your glasses, you might have two or three layers.

7. **Optional Sweetener:** Drizzle a little honey or sugar-free syrup over the top layer for added sweetness. This is optional and can be omitted for a less sweet version.

8. **Chill or Serve Immediately:** The parfait can be served immediately or chilled in the refrigerator for about 30 minutes to an hour, which allows the flavors to meld together more.

Nutritional Values (per serving)

Calories: 180, Protein: 10g, Carbohydrates: 25g, Fat: 5g, Fiber: 3g, Sodium: 50mg

Macronutrient Breakdown

Protein: 22%, Carbohydrates: 56%, Fat: 22%

Recipe Tips:

- Use fresh, crisp apples for the best flavor and texture.
- Choose low-sugar granola to maintain a low glycemic index. Be mindful of any added sugars in the granola.

Allergy Alert:

- Contains dairy and nuts (if granola includes nuts). For a nut-free version, choose nut-free granola.

Substitutions for Vegans: Use plant-based yogurt.

Substitutions for Gluten Intolerance: Use gluten-free granola.

Roasted Chickpeas

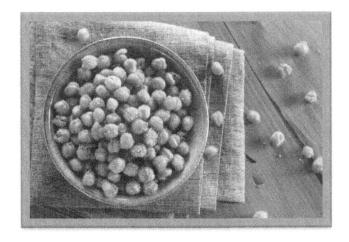

Recipe Description

Roasted Chickpeas are a crunchy and savory snack, ideal for seniors. This simple yet flavorful treat is high in protein and fiber, making it a healthy and diabetic-friendly option for a quick snack.

Preparation Time: 10 min

Cooking Time: 25 min

Servings: 4

Glycemic Index: Low

Ingredients:

- 1 can chickpeas (garbanzo beans), drained and rinsed
- 2 tablespoons olive oil
- 1 teaspoon smoked paprika
- 1/2 teaspoon garlic powder
- Salt and pepper to taste

Directions

1. **Preheat the Oven:** Preheat your oven to 400°F (200°C). This high temperature is crucial for achieving the crispy texture of the roasted chickpeas.
2. **Dry the Chickpeas:** Spread them on a clean kitchen towel or paper towel after draining and rinsing them. Pat them dry thoroughly. Removing as much moisture as possible is key to getting them nice and crispy.
3. **Season the Chickpeas:** In a mixing bowl, combine the dried chickpeas with olive oil, smoked paprika, and garlic powder. Toss them until they are evenly coated. Season with salt and pepper to your taste. The oil helps the spices stick to the chickpeas and also aids in crisping them up during roasting.
4. **Prepare for Roasting:** Spread the seasoned chickpeas in a single layer on a baking sheet. Try to ensure that the chickpeas are not overcrowded or piled on top of each other, which could prevent them from roasting evenly.
5. **Roasting Time:** Place the baking sheet in the preheated oven. Roast the chickpeas

for about 25 minutes. Halfway through, gently shake the baking sheet or use a spatula to turn the chickpeas. This helps them roast evenly and become crispy all around.

6. **Cool and Serve:** Once the chickpeas are golden and crispy, remove them from the oven. Let them cool for a few minutes; they will continue to crisp up as they cool down. Serve them as a crunchy snack.

7. **Storage:** Store the cooled chickpeas in an airtight container if you have leftovers. They can be kept for up to a week but are best when fresh.

Nutritional Values (per serving)
Calories: 150, Protein: 5g, Carbohydrates: 18g, Fat: 7g, Fiber: 5g, Sodium: 300mg
Macronutrient Breakdown
Protein: 13%, Carbohydrates: 48%, Fat: 39%

Recipe Tips:
- Make sure the chickpeas are thoroughly dried for maximum crispiness.
- Feel free to experiment with different spices and herbs for variety. Try cumin, chili powder, or a mix of herbs for different flavors.

Allergy Alert:
- No major allergens. Suitable for most dietary needs.

Substitutions for Vegans: No substitutions are needed; the recipe is already vegan.

Substitutions for Gluten Intolerance: No substitutions are needed; the recipe is gluten-free.

Baked Apple Chips

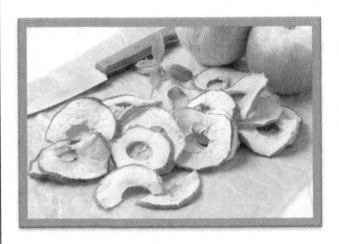

Recipe Description
Baked Apple Chips are a sweet and healthy snack, perfect for seniors. These chips are easy to make and provide a delicious, crunchy alternative to traditional snacks. They are naturally sweet, making them a great diabetic-friendly treat.

Preparation Time: 10 min
Cooking Time: 2 hours
Servings: 4
Glycemic Index: Low

Ingredients:
- 2 large apples (like Fuji or Honeycrisp)
- Cinnamon (optional)

Directions
1. **Preheat Your Oven:** Start by setting your oven to a temperature of 200°F (95°C). This low temperature will dehydrate the apples slowly, turning them into chips without burning them.
2. **Prepare the Apples:** Wash the apples thoroughly. Carefully slice the apples as thinly as possible using a mandoline or a sharp knife. Uniform, thin slices will ensure even baking and crispiness.

Remove any seeds or hard parts from the slices.

3. **Line Your Baking Sheet:** Cover a baking sheet with parchment paper. This will prevent the apple slices from sticking to the baking sheet and make cleanup easier.

4. **Arrange Apple Slices:** Place the apple slices in a single layer on the baking sheet. Avoid overlapping the slices to ensure they bake evenly and become crispy.

5. **Add Cinnamon for Flavor:** Lightly sprinkle cinnamon over the apple slices. This step is optional but adds a nice flavor to your apple chips.

6. **Bake the Apple Slices:** Place the baking sheet in the preheated oven. Bake the apple slices for 1 hour.

7. **Flip the Slices:** After 1 hour, take the baking sheet out of the oven and carefully flip each apple slice over. This will help them dry out and crisp up evenly on both sides.

8. **Finish Baking:** Return the baking sheet to the oven and bake for another hour. The extended baking time at a low temperature is key to perfect crispness.

9. **Cool the Apple Chips:** After baking, turn off the oven and let the apple chips cool inside. As they cool, they will continue to crisp up.

10. **Ready to Enjoy:** Once cooled, your apple chips will be enjoyed. Serve them as a snack anytime.

Nutritional Values (per serving)

Calories: 50, Protein: 0g, Carbohydrates: 13g, Fat: 0g, Fiber: 2g, Sodium: 0mg

Macronutrient Breakdown

Protein: 0%, Carbohydrates: 100%, Fat: 0%

Recipe Tips:

- Using a mandoline ensures evenly thin slices, which will bake more consistently.
- The apple chips can be stored in an airtight container for a few days, retaining their crispness.

Allergy Alert:

- No major allergens. Suitable for most dietary needs.

Substitutions for Vegans: No substitutions are needed; the recipe is already vegan.

Substitutions for Gluten Intolerance: No substitutions are needed; the recipe is gluten-free.

Peanut Butter and Banana Roll-Ups

Recipe Description

Peanut Butter and Banana Roll-Ups are delightful and easy-to-make snacks for seniors. Combining the creamy texture of peanut butter with the natural sweetness of bananas, these roll-ups are both nutritious and diabetic-friendly.

Preparation Time: 10 min

Cooking Time: 0 min

Servings: 4

Glycemic Index: Low to Medium

Ingredients:

- 4 whole wheat tortillas
- 1/2 cup peanut butter
- 2 bananas, sliced

- 1 tablespoon honey or sugar-free syrup (optional)
- A sprinkle of cinnamon (optional)

Directions

1. **Prepare the Ingredients::** Start by gathering all your **Ingredients:**. If the peanut butter is refrigerated, let it sit at room temperature for a few minutes to soften for easier spreading.

2. **Prepare the Tortillas:** Lay the whole wheat tortillas on a clean, flat surface like a cutting board. If the tortillas are stiff, warm them in the microwave for 10-15 seconds to make them more pliable.

3. **Spread Peanut Butter:** Take about 2 tablespoons of peanut butter for each tortilla and spread it evenly across the entire surface of each tortilla. Aim for a thin layer to avoid making the roll-ups too heavy or difficult to eat.

4. **Add Banana Slices:** Peel and slice the bananas. Arrange the banana slices in a single layer on the peanut butter. Please place them in a line down the middle or evenly across the tortilla.

5. **Add Optional Sweeteners and Cinnamon:** Drizzle a little honey or sugar-free syrup over the bananas for extra sweetness. A light sprinkle of cinnamon can also add a nice flavor, especially if you're using honey.

6. **Roll Up the Tortillas:** Carefully roll up each tortilla tightly, starting from one edge and rolling towards the opposite edge to enclose the fillings.

7. **Cut the Roll-Ups:** Using a sharp knife, cut each roll-up in half, or if preferred, slice them into bite-sized pieces for easier snacking.

8. **Serving:** The Peanut Butter and Banana Roll-Ups can be served immediately. If you prefer chilled, refrigerate them for about 30 minutes before serving.

Nutritional Values (per serving)

Calories: 300, Protein: 10g, Carbohydrates: 40g, Fat: 14g, Fiber: 5g, Sodium: 300mg

Macronutrient Breakdown

Protein: 13%, Carbohydrates: 53%, Fat: 34%

Recipe Tips:

- Using natural peanut butter without added sugars is a healthier option.
- The bananas provide natural sweetness, making additional sweeteners optional but a nice touch if a sweeter snack is desired.

Allergy Alert:

- Contains peanuts and wheat. For a peanut-free version, use almond or sunflower seed butter.

Substitutions for Vegans: No substitutions are needed if vegan-friendly tortillas and peanut butter are used.

Substitutions for Gluten Intolerance: Use gluten free tortillas.

Cottage Cheese and Fruit Bowl

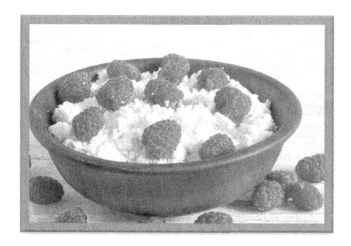

Recipe Description

The Cottage Cheese and Fruit Bowl is a refreshing and nutritious snack for seniors. This simple combination of creamy cottage cheese with fresh, sweet fruit offers a balanced snack high in protein and is suitable for a diabetic-friendly diet.

Preparation Time: 5 min

Cooking Time: 0 min

Servings: 4

Glycemic Index: Low

Ingredients:

- 2 cups low-fat cottage cheese
- 1 cup mixed fresh fruit (such as berries, peach slices, or melon cubes)
- 1 tablespoon honey or sugar-free syrup (optional)
- A sprinkle of cinnamon (optional)

Directions

1. **Prepare the Fruit:** Begin by washing the fruit thoroughly. If you're using larger fruits like peaches or melons, cut them into bite-sized cubes or slices. Berries can be used whole or halved, depending on their size.
2. **Divide the Cottage Cheese:** Evenly distribute the cottage cheese among four serving bowls. As a guideline, you can use about 1/2 cup of cottage cheese per bowl.
3. **Top with Fruit:** Arrange the prepared fruit on top of the cottage cheese in each bowl. You can create a pattern or scatter the fruit for a casual look.
4. **Add Optional Sweeteners and Spices:** Drizzle each bowl with a teaspoon of honey or sugar-free syrup for added sweetness. A light sprinkle of cinnamon can also enhance the flavor, especially with apples or peaches.
5. **Ready to Serve:** Once assembled, the Cottage Cheese and Fruit Bowls are ready to be enjoyed. They're best served fresh.

Nutritional Values (per serving)

Calories: 120, Protein: 15g, Carbohydrates: 10g, Fat: 2.5g, Fiber: 1g, Sodium: 350mg

Macronutrient Breakdown

Protein: 50%, Carbohydrates: 33%, Fat: 17%

Recipe Tips:

- Choose a variety of colorful fruits for added visual appeal and nutritional value.
- Cottage cheese is a great source of protein and calcium, making it an excellent snack option for seniors.

Allergy Alert:

- Contains dairy. For a dairy-free version, use plant-based yogurt.

Substitutions for Vegans: Use plant-based yogurt instead of cottage cheese.

Substitutions for Gluten Intolerance: No substitutions are needed; the recipe is gluten-free.

Vegetable Hummus Dip

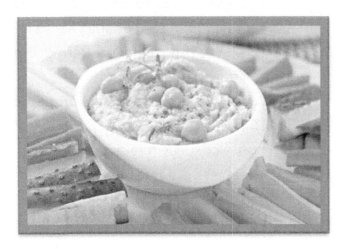

Recipe Description

Vegetable Hummus Dip is a healthy and flavorful snack, ideal for seniors. This snack combines the creamy texture of hummus with crisp, fresh vegetables for dipping, creating a nutritious and diabetic-friendly option perfect for an afternoon treat.

Preparation Time: 10 min

Cooking Time: 0 min

Servings: 4

Glycemic Index: Low

Ingredients:

- 1 cup hummus (store-bought or homemade)
- 1 cucumber, sliced
- 1 bell pepper, sliced
- 1 carrot, peeled and sliced
- 1 celery stalk, sliced

Directions

1. **Prepare the Vegetables:** Begin by washing and preparing the vegetables. Slice the cucumber and bell pepper into thin strips, peel the carrot and cut into thin slices, and slice the celery stalk. These will be your dippers for the hummus.
2. **Serving the Dip:** Scoop the hummus into a central serving bowl. Hummus can be either store-bought for convenience or homemade for a fresher taste.
3. **Arranging the Plate:** Arrange the sliced vegetables neatly around the bowl of hummus. You can organize them in groups or mix them for a colorful presentation.
4. **Ready to Serve:** Place the hummus and vegetable plate on the table. It's ready to be enjoyed as a healthy and satisfying snack.

Nutritional Values (per serving)

Calories: 150, Protein: 6g, Carbohydrates: 18g, Fat: 7g, Fiber: 5g, Sodium: 300mg

Macronutrient Breakdown

Protein: 16%, Carbohydrates: 48%, Fat: 36%

Recipe Tips:

- Making your hummus? Blend chickpeas, tahini, lemon juice, garlic, and olive oil in a food processor until smooth.
- For a colorful and nutrient-rich snack, use a variety of vegetables.

Allergy Alert:

- Hummus typically contains sesame (tahini). For a sesame-free version, look for or make a tahini-free hummus.

Substitutions for Vegans: No substitutions are needed; the recipe is already vegan.

Substitutions for Gluten Intolerance: No substitutions are needed; the recipe is gluten-free.

Whole Grain Crackers with Cheese and Tomato

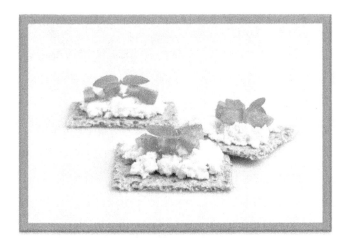

Recipe Description

Whole Grain Crackers with Cheese and Tomato perfectly balance crunchy, creamy, and fresh flavors. This simple snack, combining nutritious whole grain crackers, low-fat cheese, and ripe tomatoes, is ideal for seniors. It's an easy-to-make treat that fits well into a diabetic-friendly diet.

Preparation Time: 5 min

Cooking Time: 0 min

Servings: 4

Glycemic Index: Low to Medium

Ingredients:

- 16 whole-grain crackers
- 4 slices of low-fat cheese (such as cheddar or Swiss)
- 1 tomato, sliced
- A sprinkle of dried basil or oregano (optional)

Enhanced **Directions**

1. Prepare the **Ingredients:**:
   - Begin by slicing the tomato into thin, even slices. Aim for slices about 1/4 inch thick to sit nicely on the crackers without making them soggy.
   - If using a block of cheese, slice it into thin pieces that will fit the size of your crackers. For pre-sliced cheese, you may cut each slice into smaller pieces that match the size of the crackers.
2. Assemble the Crackers:
   - Lay your whole-grain crackers on a clean, flat surface like a cutting board or large plate.
   - Place a slice (or a piece) of cheese on each cracker. If the cheese is larger than the cracker, fold or cut it to fit so it doesn't hang over the edges.
3. Add the Tomato:
   - Top each cheese-covered cracker with a slice of tomato. Center the tomato slice to ensure each bite includes all the flavors.
   - If the tomato slices are quite juicy, you might want to gently pat them with a paper towel before placing them on the cheese to prevent the crackers from becoming soggy.
4. Seasoning:
   - Sprinkle a small amount of dried basil or oregano over the tomato

slices for added flavor. This step is optional but can enhance the overall taste of the snack.

5. Serving:
   - Serve the crackers immediately after assembly to maintain their crunchiness.
   - Arrange them nicely on a serving plate, alternating the position for a visually appealing presentation.

Nutritional Values (per serving)

Calories: 150, Protein: 6g, Carbohydrates: 15g, Fat: 8g, Fiber: 2g, Sodium: 200mg

Macronutrient Breakdown

Protein: 16%, Carbohydrates: 40%, Fat: 44%

Recipe Tips:

- Opt for whole grain crackers rich in fiber for a more nutritious snack.
- Experiment with different types of low-fat cheese like mozzarella or gouda for variety in flavor and texture.

Allergy Alert:

- Contains wheat and dairy. Use gluten-free crackers for a gluten-free option.

Substitutions

- For Vegans: Replace cheese with a vegan cheese alternative.
- For Gluten Intolerance: Opt for gluten-free crackers.

Mini Veggie Frittatas

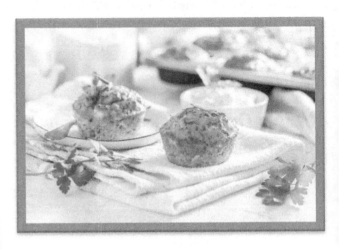

Recipe Description

Mini Veggie Frittatas are a delightful and nutritious snack or breakfast option for seniors. These individual frittatas are filled with various vegetables and baked to perfection, offering a convenient and diabetic-friendly choice.

Preparation Time: 15 min

Cooking Time: 20 min

Servings: 4 (2 mini frittatas per serving)

Glycemic Index: Low

Ingredients:

- 4 large eggs
- 1/2 cup milk
- 1/2 cup diced bell peppers
- 1/2 cup chopped spinach
- 1/4 cup diced onion
- 1/4 cup shredded low-fat cheese
- Salt and pepper to taste
- Non-stick cooking spray

Directions

1. **Preheat Oven:** Preheat your oven to 350°F (175°C). This ensures a consistent temperature for baking the frittatas.
2. **Prepare Vegetables:** Dice the bell peppers and onion, and chop the spinach

You can vary the vegetables according to your preference or your availability.

3. **Whisk Eggs and Milk:** In a large bowl, crack the eggs and add the milk. Whisk them together until fully combined. This will be the base of your frittatas.

4. **Add Vegetables and Cheese:** To the egg mixture, add the diced bell peppers, chopped spinach, diced onion, and shredded cheese. Stir to distribute the vegetables and cheese evenly. Season with salt and pepper to your liking.

5. **Prepare Muffin Tin:** Spray a muffin tin with non-stick cooking spray. This prevents the frittatas from sticking and makes them easier to remove after baking.

6. **Fill Muffin Cups:** Pour the egg and vegetable mixture into the muffin cups, filling each about 3/4 full. This allows some room for the frittatas to rise without spilling over.

7. **Bake:** Place the muffin tin in the oven for about 20 minutes. You'll know they're done when the frittatas are set and slightly golden on top.

8. **Cool and Serve:** Remove the muffin tin from the oven and let the mini frittatas cool for a few minutes. This makes them easier to handle and enjoy. Serve warm.

Nutritional Values (per serving)

Calories: 150, Protein: 10g, Carbohydrates: 5g, Fat: 10g, Fiber: 1g, Sodium: 200mg

Macronutrient Breakdown

Protein: 27%, Carbohydrates: 13%, Fat: 60%

Recipe Tips:

- You can customize these mini frittatas with different vegetables and herbs or add a bit of cooked ham or bacon for extra flavor.
- Leftovers can be stored in the refrigerator and are great for a quick snack or breakfast on the go.

Allergy Alert:

- Contains eggs and dairy. For a dairy-free version, omit the cheese or use a dairy-free alternative.

Substitutions for Vegans: Replace eggs with a vegan egg substitute, omit the cheese, or use a vegan cheese alternative.

Substitutions for Gluten Intolerance: This recipe is naturally gluten-free.

CHAPTER 6: DELICIOUS SWEETS AND DESSERTS

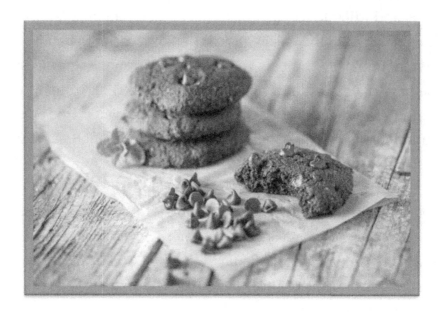

1. Classic Baked Apple Crisp

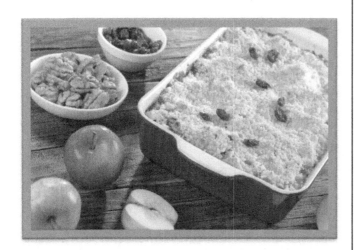

Recipe Description

This modified version of Baked Apple Crisp is ideal for seniors with diabetes, featuring a lower glycemic impact. It combines the natural sweetness of apples with a fiber-rich oat topping, using diabetic-friendly sweeteners.

Preparation Time: 15 min

Cooking Time: 45 min

Servings: 4

Glycemic Index: Low

Ingredients:

- 4 large apples, peeled, cored, and sliced
- 1/2 cup erythritol or stevia (or a blend of both)
- 1/2 cup whole wheat flour or almond flour
- 1/2 cup rolled oats
- 1/4 cup plant-based butter substitute, softened
- 1 teaspoon cinnamon
- 1/2 teaspoon nutmeg

Directions

1. **Preheat Oven:** Set your oven to 350°F (175°C).
2. **Prepare Apples:** Place the apple slices in a baking dish. Sprinkle with cinnamon and nutmeg for flavor enhancement.
3. **Make the Topping:** Combine erythritol (or stevia), whole wheat (or almond) flour

and rolled oats in a bowl. Blend in the plant-based butter until the mixture resembles coarse crumbs.

4. **Assemble:** Evenly distribute the oat mixture over the apples.

5. **Bake:** Cook in the oven for about 45 minutes. The topping should be golden brown, and the apples should be tender.

6. **Serve:** Allow cooling slightly before serving. It's great as is or with a dollop of sugar-free whipped cream.

Nutritional Values (per serving)

- Calories: 200 (approximation)
- Protein: 3g
- Carbohydrates: 30g (mostly from apples)
- Fat: 7g
- Fiber: 6g
- Sodium: 50mg

Macronutrient Breakdown

- Protein: 6%
- Carbohydrates: 60% (lower impact due to fiber and sugar substitutes)
- Fat: 34%

Recipe Tips:

- Select a mix of sweet and tart apples for a natural depth of flavor.
- Almond flour adds nuttiness and reduces carbs.

Allergy Alert:

- Contains tree nuts (if almond flour is used) and wheat (if whole wheat flour is used). Ensure that the oats and flour used are certified gluten-free for a gluten-free version.

Substitutions for Vegans: The recipe is already suitable for vegans.

2. Vanilla Brown Rice Pudding

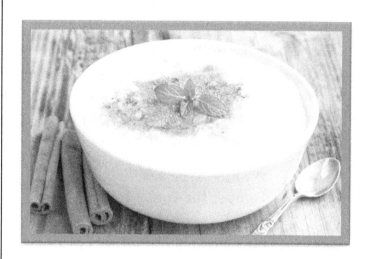

Recipe Description

Vanilla Brown Rice Pudding is a healthier twist on the classic comfort dessert. Using whole-grain brown rice and a sugar substitute, this dish is diabetic-friendly, maintaining a creamy texture and the warm vanilla essence, perfect for a sweet treat.

Preparation Time: 5 min

Cooking Time: 50 min

Servings: 4

Glycemic Index: Low to Medium

Ingredients:

- 1/2 cup uncooked brown rice
- 2 cups low-fat milk divided
- 1/3 cup sugar substitute (e.g., Stevia or Erythritol)
- 1/4 teaspoon salt
- 1 egg, beaten
- 2/3 cup golden raisins (optional; see tip below)
- 1 tablespoon unsalted butter
- 1/2 teaspoon vanilla extract

Directions

1. **Cook the Rice:** In a medium saucepan, combine the brown rice and 1 1/2 cups of milk. Cook over medium heat until the milk is mostly absorbed, about 40-45 minutes. Stir occasionally to prevent sticking.
2. **Add Sugar Substitute and Salt:** Mix the sugar and salt with the rice. Stir well to ensure it's well integrated.
3. **Temper the Egg:** Whisk the beaten egg with the remaining 1/2 cup of milk in a separate bowl. Gradually add a spoonful of the hot rice mixture to the egg mixture to temper it, preventing the egg from scrambling when added back.
4. **Combine and Cook:** Pour the tempered egg mixture into the saucepan with the rice. Cook for another 10 minutes on low heat, stirring constantly. The pudding will start to thicken.
5. **Add Flavorings:** Stir in the vanilla extract and butter until well combined. If using raisins, consider adding them now, or see the recipe tip below.
6. **Serve:** Spoon the rice pudding into bowls. It can be enjoyed warm or chilled. Refrigerate any leftovers.

Nutritional Values (per serving)

- Calories: 180
- Protein: 6g
- Carbohydrates: 30g (complex)
- Fat: 4g
- Fiber: 2g
- Sodium: 100mg

Macronutrient Breakdown

- Protein: 13%
- Carbohydrates: 67%
- Fat: 20%

Recipe Tips:

- **Raisins:** If added, use a smaller amount to limit the sugar content, or consider using fresh berries as a substitute for a lower glycemic impact.
- **Stirring:** Frequent stirring ensures a smooth texture without sticking or burning.
- **Brown Rice:** Using brown rice adds fiber and nutrients compared to white rice, making it a healthier choice for blood sugar management.

Allergy Alert:

- Contains dairy and egg. For dairy-free, use almond or soy milk.

Substitutions for Vegans: Replace the dairy milk with a plant-based alternative and use a vegan egg substitute.

This recipe modification aims to make the dessert more suitable for individuals managing diabetes by incorporating whole grains, reducing simple sugars, and maintaining a balance of macronutrients.

Peach Cobbler with Cinnamon Crust

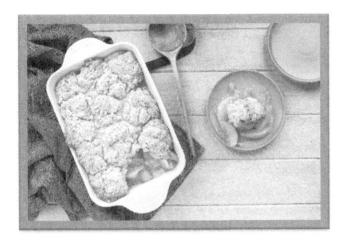

Recipe Description:
This adapted Peach Cobbler is suitable for people with diabetes and features low-glycemic sweeteners and whole-grain flour. The cinnamon-spiced crust adds a delightful touch to this healthy and flavorful dessert.

Preparation Time: 10 min
Cooking Time: 35 min
Servings: 4
Glycemic Index: Low to Medium

Ingredients::

- 4 cups sliced peaches
- 3/4 cup Erythritol or Stevia
- 3/4 cup whole wheat flour
- 1/4 cup almond flour
- 1 tsp baking powder
- 1/2 tsp cinnamon
- 1/4 cup plant-based butter, melted
- 1/4 cup milk (dairy or plant-based)

Directions:

1. **Preheat Oven**: Set your oven to 350°F (175°C).
2. **Prepare Peaches**: In a baking dish, place the peach slices. Sprinkle them with cinnamon.
3. **Make Topping**: In a bowl, mix Erythritol (or Stevia), whole wheat flour, almond flour, and baking powder. Add melted plant-based butter and milk, stirring until just combined.
4. **Assemble Cobbler**: Spoon the topping evenly over the peaches.
5. **Bake**: Cook in the oven for about 35 minutes until the topping is golden brown and peaches are tender.
6. **Serve**: Let it cool slightly before serving. Ideal with a dollop of sugar-free whipped cream.

Nutritional Values (approximation per serving):

- Calories: 200
- Protein: 4g
- Carbohydrates: 30g
- Fat: 8g
- Fiber: 5g
- Sodium: 50mg

Macronutrient Breakdown:

- Protein: 8%
- Carbohydrates: 60%
- Fat: 32%

Recipe Tips::

- Choose a mix of sweet and tart peaches for better flavor.
- Almond flour adds a nutty taste and reduces carbs.

Allergy Alert::

- Contains tree nuts (almond flour). For a gluten-free version, ensure to use gluten-free flour.

Substitutions for Vegans:

- The recipe is suitable for vegans as is.

4. Lemon Bars with Shortbread Crust

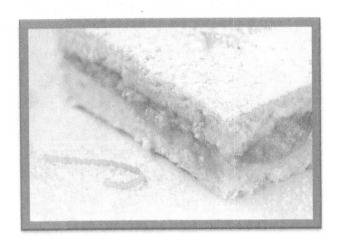

Recipe Description

These modified Lemon Bars, tailored for a diabetic-friendly diet, retain the classic American dessert's zesty flavor and delicate crust, now made with healthier **Ingredients:** suitable for managing blood sugar levels.

Preparation Time: 25 min

Cooking Time: 45 min

Servings: 4

Glycemic Index: Low

Ingredients:

- For the Shortbread Crust:
    - 1 cup almond flour (instead of all-purpose flour)
    - 1/4 cup erythritol (instead of powdered sugar)
    - 1/2 cup butter, softened (use plant-based butter for dairy-free version)
- For the Lemon Filling:
    - 2 large eggs (use a vegan egg substitute for vegans)
    - 1 cup erythritol (instead of granulated sugar)
    - 2 tablespoons coconut flour (instead of all-purpose flour)
    - 1/4 cup fresh lemon juice
    - 1 teaspoon lemon zest
    - Erythritol for dusting (instead of powdered sugar)

Directions

1. Prepare the Crust: Preheat oven to 350°F (175°C). In a bowl, mix almond flour and erythritol. Cut in the softened butter until the mixture resembles coarse crumbs. Press into the bottom of a lightly greased 8x8-inch baking dish. Bake for 25 minutes or until lightly browned.
2. Make the Lemon Filling: While the crust bakes, whisk together eggs and erythritol until smooth. Stir in coconut flour, lemon juice, and zest. Mix well.
3. Assemble and Bake: Pour lemon filling over the baked crust. Return to the oven and bake for 20 minutes or until the filling is set.
4. Cool and Serve: Let cool to room temperature. Dust with erythritol, cut into bars, and serve.

Nutritional Values (per serving)

Calories: 320, Protein: 6g, Carbohydrates: 20g, Fat: 26g, Fiber: 3g, Sodium: 120mg Macronutrient Breakdown Protein: 7%, Carbohydrates: 25%, Fat: 68%

Recipe Tips:

- Keep a close watch on the crust; almond flour can brown quickly.
- Fresh lemon juice and zest are key for vibrant flavor.

- Contains nuts and eggs. For a dairy-free version, use plant-based butter.

Substitutions for Vegans: Replace eggs with a vegan substitute and use plant-based butter. Substitutions for Gluten Intolerance: This recipe is gluten-free.

5. Old-Fashioned Bread Pudding

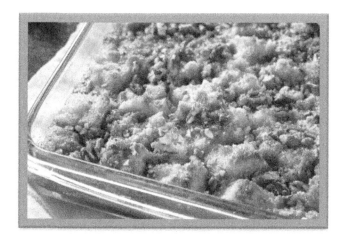

Recipe Description

This revised Old-Fashioned Bread Pudding is a comforting, homey dessert, now adapted to be more suitable for individuals managing diabetes. This version maintains the classic essence while using diabetic-friendly **Ingredients:**, transforming it into a warm, custardy treat that is lower in sugars and higher in fiber.

Preparation Time: 20 min

Cooking Time: 50 min

Servings: 4

Glycemic Index: Low

Ingredients:

- 4 cups cubed day-old whole grain bread (richer in fiber)
- 2 cups unsweetened almond milk (instead of regular milk)
- 1/4 cup butter (use plant-based butter for dairy-free)
- 1/3 cup erythritol (instead of sugar)
- 2 eggs, lightly beaten (use a vegan egg substitute for vegans)
- 1 teaspoon vanilla extract
- 1/2 teaspoon cinnamon
- 1/4 teaspoon nutmeg
- 1/2 cup fresh blueberries or chopped apples (instead of raisins)

Directions

1. Preheat and Prepare: Set the oven to 350°F (175°C). Lightly grease a baking dish.
2. Soften the Bread: Pour almond milk over the bread cubes in a large bowl. Let it sit for 10 minutes to soften.
3. Melt Butter and Erythritol: Melt the butter in a saucepan over low heat. Stir in erythritol until it dissolves.
4. Combine **Ingredients:**: Add melted butter and erythritol, beaten eggs, vanilla extract, cinnamon, nutmeg, and blueberries or apples to the bread mixture. Stir gently.
5. Transfer to Baking Dish: Pour the mixture into the prepared baking dish and spread evenly.
6. Bake for 50 minutes until the top is golden and the center is set.
7. Cool and Serve: Allow to cool slightly before serving. Enjoy warm or at room temperature.

Nutritional Values (per serving)

Calories: 300, Protein: 10g, Carbohydrates: 40g, Fat: 12g, Fiber: 5g, Sodium: 250mg

Macronutrient Breakdown

Protein 13%, Carbohydrates: 53%, Fat: 34%

Recipe Tips:

- Whole grain bread enhances fiber content, which is beneficial for blood sugar management.
- Fresh fruits add natural sweetness and additional fiber.

Allergy Alert:

- Contains wheat, eggs, and dairy (if not using substitutes). For a dairy-free version, use plant-based milk and butter.

Substitutions for Vegans: Use vegan butter, plant-based milk, and a vegan egg substitute. Substitutions for Gluten Intolerance: Use gluten-free bread.

---

6. Baked Custard with Nutmeg

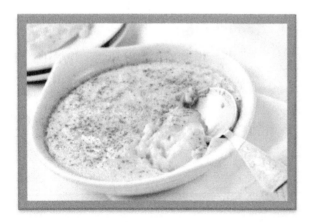

Recipe Description

This Baked Custard with Nutmeg has been adapted for a diabetic-friendly diet, maintaining its timeless appeal. The smooth, creamy texture is preserved, and the comforting taste of nutmeg remains a highlight, with adjustments made to suit the dietary needs of individuals with diabetes.

Preparation Time: 15 min

Cooking Time: 45 min

Servings: 4

Glycemic Index: Low

Ingredients:

- 4 large eggs (or vegan egg substitute)
- 1/3 cup erythritol (instead of granulated sugar)
- 1/2 teaspoon vanilla extract
- 2 1/2 cups unsweetened almond milk (or any plant-based milk)
- Ground nutmeg for sprinkling

Directions

1. Preheat the Oven: Preheat your oven to 325°F (165°C).
2. Prepare Water Bath: Fill a large baking dish halfway with water and place it in the oven. This is your water bath for the custard.
3. Whisk Eggs and Erythritol: In a bowl, whisk together the eggs and erythritol until well blended. Mix in the vanilla extract.
4. Heat the Milk: Gently warm the almond milk in a saucepan until it's warm but not boiling.
5. Combine and Strain: Gradually whisk the warm milk into the egg mixture. Strain through a fine sieve to remove any lumps.
6. Pour into Dishes: Evenly divide the custard mixture among 4 ramekins. Sprinkle each with ground nutmeg.

7. Bake in Water Bath: Place the ramekins in the water bath in the oven. Bake for 45 minutes until custard is set but slightly wobbly in the center.

8. Cool and Serve: Remove from the oven and water bath. Cool to room temperature, then refrigerate until chilled.

Nutritional Values (per serving)

Calories: 180, Protein: 9g, Carbohydrates: 15g, Fat: 10g, Fiber: 1g, Sodium: 90mg

Macronutrient Breakdown

Protein: 20%, Carbohydrates: 33%, Fat: 47%

Recipe Tips:

- A water bath is crucial for even gentler cooking of the custard.
- Erythritol is a sugar alcohol with minimal impact on blood sugar, making it a suitable alternative for sugar in diabetic-friendly recipes.

Allergy Alert:

- Contains eggs. For a dairy-free version, use plant-based milk.

Substitutions for Vegans: Replace eggs with a vegan egg substitute and use plant-based milk.

7. Mixed Berry Compote with Yogurt

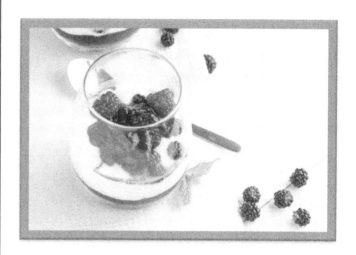

Recipe Description

This Mixed Berry Compote with Yogurt is a refreshing, light dessert now adapted for a diabetic-friendly diet. It features the natural sweetness of berries and the creamy texture of yogurt, creating a balanced and enjoyable treat for those managing diabetes.

Preparation Time: 15 min

Cooking Time: 15 min

Servings: 4

Glycemic Index: Low

Ingredients:

- 2 cups mixed berries (like strawberries, blueberries, or raspberries)
- 2 tablespoons erythritol or stevia (instead of honey or traditional sugar substitutes)
- 1 teaspoon lemon juice
- 1 cup low-fat Greek yogurt (use a plant-based yogurt for dairy-free and vegan versions)

Directions

1. Prepare the Berries: Wash and cut larger berries into smaller pieces.
2. Cook the Berries: Over medium heat, mix berries, erythritol or stevia, and lemon juice in a saucepan. Cook for about 15 minutes or until berries are soft and have released their juices.
3. Cool the Compote: After the berries soften, remove them from heat and let them cool. The compote will thicken as it cools.
4. Assemble the Dessert: Spoon Greek yogurt into bowls and top with berry compote.
5. Serve: Enjoy immediately or refrigerate. It can be served cold or at room temperature.

Nutritional Values (per serving)

Calories: 100, Protein: 6g, Carbohydrates: 18g, Fat: 1g, Fiber: 4g, Sodium: 30mg

Macronutrient Breakdown

Protein: 24%, Carbohydrates: 72%, Fat: 4%

Recipe Tips:
- Fresh berries offer the best flavor and nutrient content, but frozen berries can also be used.
- Adjust the level of sweetness with erythritol or stevia to suit your preference.

Allergy Alert:
- Contains dairy. For a dairy-free version, use a plant-based yogurt alternative.

Substitutions for Vegans:

Opt for a vegan-friendly yogurt substitute.

8. No-Bake Peanut Butter Oat Bars

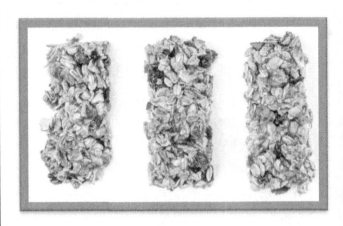

Recipe Description

These adapted No-Bake Peanut Butter Oat Bars are perfect for seniors, combining the heartiness of oats with creamy peanut butter in a diabetic-friendly format. They're simple to make, don't require baking, and are a great treat for managing blood sugar levels.

Preparation Time: 20 min

Chilling Time: 1 hour

Servings: 4

Glycemic Index: Low

Ingredients:
- 1 cup rolled oats (use whole grain oats for more fiber)
- 1/2 cup natural peanut butter (unsweetened)
- 1/4 cup sugar-free syrup (like erythritol-based syrup instead of honey)
- 1/2 teaspoon vanilla extract
- Pinch of salt

Directions
1. Mix **Ingredients:**: Combine rolled oats, peanut butter, sugar-free syrup, vanilla

extract, and a pinch of salt in a bowl. Mix until sticky and well combined.

2. Prepare the Pan: Line an 8x8 inch pan with parchment paper.

3. Press Mixture into Pan: Transfer the mixture to the pan. Press down firmly into an even layer. Smooth the surface with a spoon or hands.

4. Chill: Refrigerate for at least 1 hour or until firm.

5. Cut into Bars: Lift the mixture from the pan using parchment paper cut into bars or squares on a cutting board.

6. Serve or Store: Enjoy immediately or store in an airtight container in the refrigerator.

Nutritional Values (per serving)

Calories: 250, Protein: 9g, Carbohydrates: 28g, Fat: 13g, Fiber: 5g, Sodium: 80mg

Macronutrient Breakdown

Protein: 14%, Carbohydrates: 45%, Fat: 41%

Recipe Tips:

- Add chopped nuts or seeds for extra crunch and nutrition.
- Room-temperature peanut butter blends more easily.

Allergy Alert:

- Contains peanuts. Use almond butter or sunflower seed butter for a peanut-free version.

Substitutions for Vegans:

Ensure the sugar-free syrup is vegan-friendly.

---

9. Baked Banana Pudding

Recipe Description

Baked Banana Pudding is a classic American dessert that is especially popular among seniors. It features layers of ripe bananas, soft vanilla wafers, and a rich custard baked to perfection.

Preparation Time: 15 min

Cooking Time: 30 min

Servings: 4

Glycemic Index: Low to Medium

Ingredients:

- 3 ripe bananas, sliced
- 1/2 cup granulated sugar
- 2 cups milk
- 3 tablespoons all-purpose flour
- 1/4 teaspoon salt
- 2 large eggs, separated
- 1 teaspoon vanilla extract
- 1/2 cup vanilla wafers

Directions

1. **Preheat Oven and Prepare Dish:** Preheat your oven to 350°F (175°C). Lightly grease a baking dish.

2. **Layer Bananas and Wafers:** Arrange a layer of vanilla wafers at the bottom of the dish. Top with a layer of sliced bananas.

3. **Make Custard:** In a saucepan, combine sugar, flour, and salt. Gradually stir in the milk. Cook over medium heat, stirring constantly, until thickened. Remove from heat.

4. **Temper Egg Yolks:** Beat the egg yolks in a separate bowl. Gradually whisk in a small amount of the hot custard to temper the yolks. Then, slowly whisk the tempered yolks back into the saucepan with the custard.

5. **Cook Custard with Yolks:** Cook the custard over low heat for two minutes, stirring constantly. Remove from heat and stir in vanilla extract.

6. **Assemble Pudding:** Pour the custard over the bananas and wafers in the baking dish.

7. **Bake:** Bake for 15 minutes.

8. **Make Meringue (Optional):** Beat the egg whites until stiff peaks form. Gradually add 1/4 cup sugar, beating until glossy. Spread the meringue over the pudding.

9. **Brown Meringue:** Return to the oven and bake for 15 minutes or until the meringue is lightly browned.

10. **Cool and Serve:** Allow the pudding to cool slightly before serving. It can be enjoyed warm or chilled.

Nutritional Values (per serving)

Calories: 300, Protein: 7g, Carbohydrates: 50g, Fat: 8g, Fiber: 2g, Sodium: 200mg

Macronutrient Breakdown

Protein: 9%, Carbohydrates: 67%, Fat: 24%

Recipe Tips:

- Ensure the bananas are ripe for the best flavor.
- The meringue topping is optional but adds a delightful lightness and visual appeal to the dessert.

Allergy Alert:

- Contains wheat, eggs, and dairy. For a dairy-free version, use almond or soy milk.

Substitutions for Vegans: Use plant-based milk, egg substitutes, and vegan wafers.

11.   Cinnamon-Spiced Baked Pears

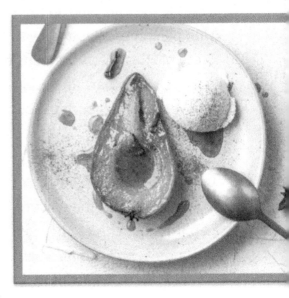

12.

Recipe Description

In this diabetic-friendly adaptation, Cinnamon-spiced baked Pears offer a subtle sweetness and warm spice, perfect for seniors. This dessert emphasizes the natural flavors of pears, enhanced with cinnamon, without added sugars

Preparation Time: 15 min

Cooking Time: 30 min

Servings: 4

Glycemic Index: Low

Ingredients:

- 4 ripe pears, halved and cored
- 2 tablespoons erythritol (instead of brow sugar)
- 1/2 teaspoon ground cinnamon
- 1/4 teaspoon ground nutmeg
- 2 tablespoons butter, cut into small pieces (use plant-based butter for dairy-free)
- Optional: Sugar-free vanilla ice cream or whipped cream for serving

Directions

1. Preheat the oven: Set it to 375°F (190 °C).
2. Prepare Pears: Slice pears in half, remove cores, and place them cut side up in a baking dish.
3. Mix Erythritol and Spices: Combine erythritol, cinnamon, and nutmeg. Sprinkle over pears.
4. Add Butter: Place a small piece of butter on each pear half. This helps in caramelization during baking.
5. Bake: Bake for 30 minutes until pears are soft, and the tops are caramelized.
6. Serve: Cool slightly. Serve warm, alone or with sugar-free vanilla ice cream or whipped cream.

Nutritional Values (per serving)

Calories: 130, Protein: 1g, Carbohydrates: 27g, Fat: 4g, Fiber: 6g, Sodium: 40mg

Macronutrient Breakdown

Protein: 3%, Carbohydrates: 75%, Fat: 22%

Recipe Tips:

- Ripe but firm pears are ideal for maintaining texture during baking.
- Baking times may vary slightly based on pear variety and size.

Allergy Alert:

- Contains dairy. For a dairy-free version, use plant-based butter.

Substitutions for Vegans:

Use a vegan butter substitute. Serve with vegan ice cream or coconut whipped cream if desired.

CHAPTER 7: BEVERAGES AND SMOOTHIES

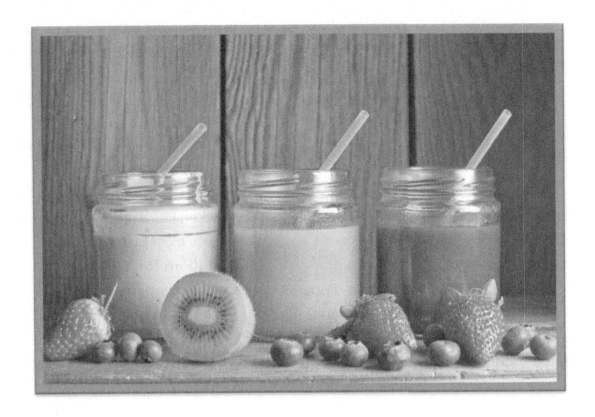

RECIPES: INCLUDE RECIPES FOR SMOOTHIES, COCKTAILS, AND OTHER DRINKS.

Do you need low-calorie cocktails, coffee beverages, smoothies, and shakes? You've arrived at the ideal location!

Anyone can make smoothies, cocktails, and other healthy drink ideas, and they have fewer calories and sugar than their more conventional counterparts.

You can see the amount of calories and other nutritional info in every dish, making them ideal for weight reduction and control!

1. Classic Hot Lemon and Honey Tea

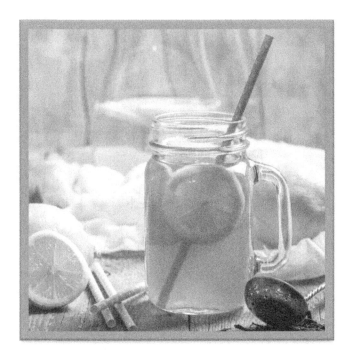

Recipe Description

This Hot Lemon and Low-Glycemic Sweetener Tea offers a comforting and healthful beverage for seniors. Using a low-glycemic sweetener makes it suitable for those managing diabetes, while the lemon adds a refreshing zest.

Preparation Time: 5 min

Cooking Time: 0 min

Servings: 1

Glycemic Index: Low

Ingredients:

- 1 cup hot water
- 1 tablespoon low-glycemic sweetener (such as stevia or erythritol)
- 2 tablespoons fresh lemon juice
- Optional: a slice of lemon for garnish

Directions

1. **Heat the Water:** Boil water in a kettle or on the stove. Once boiled, let it cool for about a minute to avoid overheating the sweetener and lemon juice.
2. **Prepare the Tea:** Add the low-glycemic sweetener and fresh lemon juice to a cup. Pour the hot water over these **Ingredients:**, ensuring the sweetener dissolves completely.
3. **Garnish and Serve:** Optionally, garnish with a slice of lemon on the cup's rim for added flavor and presentation. Serve the tea while it's warm to enjoy its soothing effects.

Nutritional Values (approx. per serving)

- Calories: negligible
- Protein: 0g
- Carbohydrates: negligible
- Fat: 0g
- Fiber: 0g
- Sodium: negligible

Macronutrient Breakdown

- Protein: 0%
- Carbohydrates: negligible
- Fat: 0%

Recipe Tips:

- Adjust the amount of sweetener and lemon juice to taste.
- This beverage is ideal for cold days or soothing relaxation.

Allergy Alert:

- No known allergens. Suitable for most dietary needs.

2. Classic Banana Smoothie

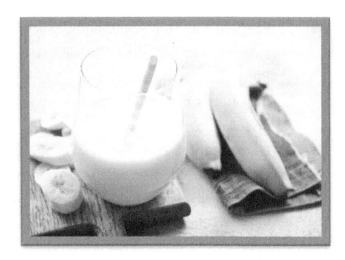

Recipe Description

A Classic Banana Smoothie is a nutritious and delicious beverage, perfect for seniors. It's a great way to incorporate fruit into the diet, offering natural sweetness and a creamy texture.

Preparation Time: 5 min

Cooking Time: 0 min

Servings: 1

Glycemic Index: Low to Medium

Ingredients:

- 1 ripe banana
- 1 cup milk (dairy or plant-based)
- 1/2 cup plain yogurt (optional for extra creaminess)
- 1 tablespoon honey or a sugar substitute (optional)
- A few ice cubes (optional)

Directions

1. **Prepare the Banana:** Peel the ripe banana and break it into chunks. Ripe bananas add natural sweetness and creaminess to the smoothie.
2. **Blend Ingredients::** In a blender, combine the banana chunks, milk, and yogurt (if using). If you prefer a sweeter taste, add honey or a sugar substitute.
3. **Add Ice (Optional):** Add a few ice cubes to the blender for a colder and more refreshing smoothie.
4. **Blend Until Smooth:** Blend all **Ingredients:** quickly until smooth and creamy. The mixture should have a uniform consistency.
5. **Taste and Adjust:** Taste the smoothie. You can add more honey or milk to adjust the sweetness and thickness if needed.
6. **Serve Immediately:** Pour the smoothie into a glass and serve immediately for the best flavor and texture.

Nutritional Values (per serving)

Calories: 200, Protein: 8g, Carbohydrates: 35g, Fat: 4g, Fiber: 3g, Sodium: 80mg

Macronutrient Breakdown

Protein: 16%, Carbohydrates: 70%, Fat: 14%

Recipe Tips:

- Use a frozen banana for a thicker, ice cream-like texture.
- This smoothie can be customized with other fruits, such as berries or peaches, for added flavor and nutrients.

Allergy Alert:

- Contains dairy. For a dairy-free version, use plant-based milk and yogurt.

Substitutions for Vegans: Use almond, soy, or coconut milk and a vegan yogurt alternative.

3. Green Tea with Mint and Honey

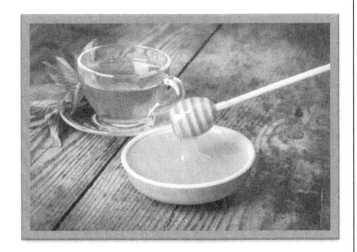

Recipe Description

Green Tea with Mint and Honey is a refreshing and healthful beverage, ideal for seniors. It combines the antioxidant properties of green tea with the soothing effects of mint and the natural sweetness of honey.

Preparation Time: 5 min

Brewing Time: 3 min

Servings: 1

Glycemic Index: Low

Ingredients:

- 1 green tea bag
- 1 cup boiling water
- A few fresh mint leaves
- 1 tablespoon honey (optional)

Directions

1. **Boil Water:** Start by boiling water in a kettle. Once boiled, let it cool for about a minute. Green tea brews best in water that's just below boiling.
2. **Prepare the Tea:** Place the green tea bag in a cup. Pour the hot water over the tea bag.
3. **Steep the Tea:** Let the tea steep for about 3 minutes. This allows the flavors to infuse without making the tea bitter.
4. **Add Mint:** While the tea is steeping, rinse a few fresh mint leaves. Add them to the cup. The heat from the tea will release the mint's flavor and aroma.
5. **Sweeten with Honey:** If desired, stir in a tablespoon of honey to add natural sweetness to the tea.
6. **Serve:** Remove the tea bag once the tea has steeped and is infused with mint. Stir well and enjoy the refreshing and soothing beverage.

Nutritional Values (per serving)

Calories: 60 (if honey is added), Protein: 0g, Carbohydrates: 17g (from honey), Fat: 0g, Fiber: 0g, Sodium: 0mg

Macronutrient Breakdown

Protein: 0%, Carbohydrates: 100% (if honey is added), Fat: 0%

Recipe Tips:

- Adjust the steeping time according to your taste preference. Less time will result in a milder flavor, while more time will increase the intensity.
- The mint leaves can be muddled before adding to the tea for a stronger mint flavor.

Allergy Alert:

- No known allergens. Suitable for most dietary needs.

Substitutions for Vegans: Honey can be replaced with agave syrup or omitted.

4. Classic Strawberry Smoothie

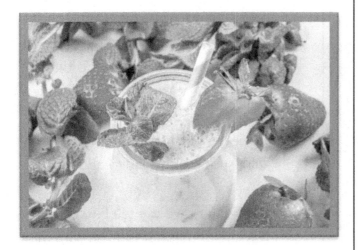

Recipe Description

A Classic Strawberry Smoothie is a delightful and nutritious drink for seniors. It's a great way to enjoy the natural sweetness of strawberries in a creamy, refreshing beverage.

Preparation Time: 5 min

Cooking Time: 0 min

Servings: 1

Glycemic Index: Low to Medium

Ingredients:

- 1 cup fresh or frozen strawberries
- 1 banana (optional for added sweetness)
- 1 cup milk (dairy or plant-based)
- 1/2 cup plain yogurt (optional for extra creaminess)
- 1 tablespoon honey or sugar substitute (optional)

Directions

1. **Prepare Ingredients::** If using fresh strawberries, wash and hull them. If you're using a banana, peel and slice it.
2. **Blend the Fruits:** Place the strawberries (and banana, if using) in a blender.
3. **Add Milk and Yogurt:** Pour in the milk and add the yogurt. The yogurt is optional but gives the smoothie a creamier texture.
4. **Sweeten if Needed:** Add honey or a sugar substitute for a sweeter smoothie. This step is optional and can be adjusted to taste.
5. **Blend Until Smooth:** Blend all **Ingredients:** on high speed until smooth. If the smoothie is too thick, add more milk to reach your desired consistency.
6. **Taste and Adjust:** Taste the smoothie and adjust sweetness or thickness.
7. **Serve Immediately:** Pour the smoothie into a glass and serve immediately for the best flavor.

Nutritional Values (per serving)

Calories: 200 (varies depending on **Ingredients:** used), Protein: 8g, Carbohydrates: 35g, Fat: 4g, Fiber: 4g, Sodium: 80mg

Macronutrient Breakdown

Protein: 16%, Carbohydrates: 70%, Fat: 14%

Recipe Tips:

- Using frozen strawberries will give the smoothie a thicker, cooler texture.
- For added flavor and nutrition, you can add other fruits like blueberries or raspberries.

Allergy Alert:

- Contains dairy. Use almond, soy, or coconut milk and a plant-based yogurt for a dairy-free version.

Substitutions for Vegans: Use a vegan-friendly sweetener and plant-based yogurt.

5. Classic Iced Tea with Lemon

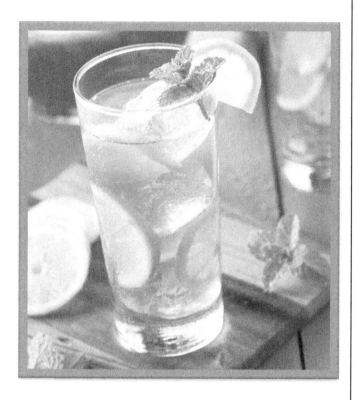

Recipe Description

Classic Iced Tea with Lemon is a refreshing and timeless beverage, particularly beloved by seniors on warm days. This simple drink combines the brisk flavors of tea with a zesty lemon twist.

Preparation Time: 10 min (plus chilling time)

Brewing Time: 5 min

Servings: 4

Glycemic Index: Low

Ingredients:

- 4 tea bags (black or green tea)
- 4 cups of water
- 2 tablespoons honey or sugar substitute (optional)
- 1 lemon, sliced
- Ice cubes
- Fresh mint leaves (optional, for garnish)

Directions

1. **Boil Water:** Start by bringing water to a boil in a kettle or pot.
2. **Steep the Tea:** Once the water is boiling, remove it from the heat and add the tea bags. Let them steep for about 5 minutes. Adjust the steeping time based on how strong you like your tea.
3. **Sweeten the Tea:** After steeping, remove the tea bags. If you add honey or a sugar substitute, do it while the tea is still warm so it dissolves easily.
4. **Cool the Tea:** Allow the tea to cool to room temperature. Then, refrigerate it until it's cold. This may take about 1-2 hours.
5. **Prepare Serving Glasses:** Fill serving glasses with ice cubes. Add a slice or two of lemon to each glass.
6. **Serve the Tea:** Pour the chilled tea over the ice. Stir gently.
7. **Garnish and Enjoy:** Garnish with a sprig of fresh mint if desired. Serve the iced tea immediately for a refreshing drink.

Nutritional Values (per serving)

Calories: 30 (if honey is added), Protein: 0g, Carbohydrates: 8g (from honey), Fat: 0g, Fiber: 0g, Sodium: 0mg

Macronutrient Breakdown

Protein: 0%, Carbohydrates: 100% (if honey is added), Fat: 0%

Recipe Tips:

- For a stronger lemon flavor, squeeze a lemon wedge into each glass before serving.
- The tea can be prepared and stored in the refrigerator for 2-3 days.

Allergy Alert:

- No known allergens. Suitable for most dietary needs.

Substitutions for Vegans: Use a vegan-friendly sweetener like agave nectar instead of honey.

---

6. Blueberry Almond Milk Smoothie

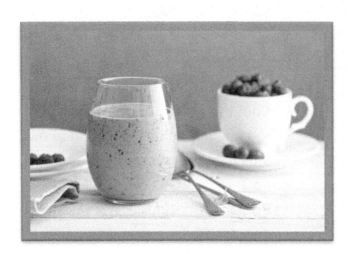

Recipe Description

The Blueberry Almond Milk Smoothie is a delightful and nutritious drink for seniors. It combines the antioxidant benefits of blueberries with the creamy texture of almond milk, creating a delicious and healthful beverage.

Preparation Time: 5 min

Cooking Time: 0 min

Servings: 1

Glycemic Index: Low

Ingredients:

- 1 cup blueberries (fresh or frozen)
- 1 banana (optional for added sweetness and creaminess)
- 1 cup unsweetened almond milk
- 1 tablespoon almond butter or ground almonds
- 1 tablespoon honey or sugar substitute (optional)

- Ice cubes (optional)

Directions

1. **Prepare the Fruits:** If you use fresh blueberries, wash them thoroughly. Peel the banana and cut it into chunks if you include it.
2. **Blend the Ingredients::** In a blender, combine the blueberries, banana, almond milk, and almond butter or ground almonds. If you prefer a sweeter smoothie, add honey or a sugar substitute.
3. **Add Ice for Texture:** Add some ice cubes to the blender for a cooler and thicker smoothie.
4. **Blend Until Smooth:** Process all the **Ingredients:** quickly until smooth. Add more almond milk to adjust the consistency if the smoothie is too thick.
5. **Taste and Adjust:** Taste the smoothie and adjust the sweetness or thickness as desired.
6. **Serve Immediately:** Pour the smoothie into a glass and enjoy it fresh for the best taste.

Nutritional Values (per serving)

Calories: 180 (varies with **Ingredients:**), Protein: 4g, Carbohydrates: 30g, Fat: 6g, Fiber: 5g, Sodium: 60mg

Macronutrient Breakdown

Protein: 9%, Carbohydrates: 67%, Fat: 24%

Recipe Tips:

- Using frozen blueberries will give the smoothie a chilled, ice-cream-like consistency.

- You can add a handful of spinach for extra nutrition without altering the taste significantly.

Allergy Alert:
- Contains nuts. For those allergic to almonds, substitute with another type of milk and nut butter.

Substitutions for Vegans: This recipe is already vegan-friendly.

7. Warm Spiced Apple Cider

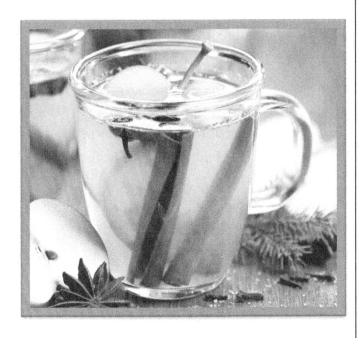

Recipe Description: This Warm Spiced Apple Cider is a comforting beverage for seniors, especially during cooler seasons. Modified to fit ADA guidelines, it uses unsweetened apple cider and a sugar substitute, combining warm spices for a delightful drink.

Preparation Time: 5 min
Cooking Time: 15 min
Servings: 4
Glycemic Index: Low

Ingredients::
- 4 cups unsweetened apple cider
- 2 cinnamon sticks
- 4 cloves
- 2 star anise
- 1 orange, sliced
- 1 tablespoon sugar substitute (such as stevia or erythritol)
- Optional: Additional cinnamon sticks for garnish

Directions:
1. **Combine Ingredients::** In a large pot, combine the unsweetened apple cider, cinnamon sticks, cloves, star anise, and orange slices.
2. **Simmer:** Place the pot over medium heat and bring the mixture to a low simmer. Avoid boiling to maintain the delicate flavors of the spices.
3. **Infuse the Flavors:** Let the cider simmer gently for about 15 minutes. This allows the spices and orange flavors to infuse into the cider.
4. **Sweeten:** If desired, add a tablespoon of a sugar substitute to enhance the sweetness without raising the glycemic index.
5. **Serve Warm:** Once the cider is infused, remove it from heat. Spoon the warm cider into mugs or cups, leaving the solid **Ingredients:** behind.
6. **Garnish:** If you like, garnish each serving with an additional cinnamon stick for a festive touch.
7. **Enjoy:** Serve the spiced apple cider warm, enjoying the aromatic blend of flavors.

Nutritional Values (approximation per serving):

- Calories: 120 (varies based on the specific sugar substitute used)
- Protein: 0g
- Carbohydrates: 30g (natural sugars from apples)
- Fat: 0g
- Fiber: 1g
- Sodium: 10mg

Macronutrient Breakdown:

- Protein: 0%
- Carbohydrates: 100%
- Fat: 0%

Recipe Tips::

- For a stronger flavor, simmer the cider longer, allowing more time for the spices to infuse.
- This recipe can be easily scaled up for larger gatherings.

Allergy Alert::

- Suitable for most dietary needs.

Substitutions for Vegans:

- No substitutions are needed; the recipe is already vegan-friendly.

8. Cucumber and Mint Infused Water

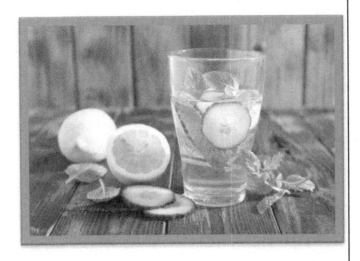

Recipe Description: This Cucumber and Mint Infused Water is an excellent hydrating option for seniors. It's incredibly simple to prepare and offers a subtle, refreshing flavor, making it an ideal beverage for all-day hydration.

Preparation Time: 5 min (plus infusing time)

Cooking Time: 0 min

Servings: 4

Glycemic Index: Low

Ingredients::

- 1 large cucumber, thinly sliced
- A handful of fresh mint leaves
- 4 cups of water
- Ice cubes (optional)

Directions:

1. **Prepare the Ingredients::** Wash the cucumber thoroughly and slice it thinly. Clean the mint leaves to remove any dirt or debris.
2. **Infuse the Water:** Add the sliced cucumber and fresh mint leaves in a large pitcher. Fill the pitcher with 4 cups of water.
3. **Chill and Infuse:** Refrigerate the pitcher for at least 1 hour to allow the flavors of the cucumber and mint to infuse the water. For a more pronounced flavor, you can leave it longer, even overnight.
4. **Serve:** To serve, fill glasses with ice cubes (if using) and pour the infused water over them.
5. **Garnish:** Add a few extra cucumber slices and a sprig of mint to each glass for added visual appeal and flavor.
6. **Enjoy:** Sip this light and refreshing beverage throughout the day.

Nutritional Values (per serving):

- Calories: Negligible
- Protein: 0g
- Carbohydrates: 0g
- Fat: 0g
- Fiber: 0g
- Sodium: 0mg

Macronutrient Breakdown:

- Protein: 0%
- Carbohydrates: 0%
- Fat: 0%

Recipe Tips::

- The quantity of cucumber and mint can be adjusted based on personal preference.
- This drink is an excellent way to stay hydrated, particularly for those who might not enjoy plain water.

Allergy Alert::

- No known allergens. Suitable for all dietary needs.

Substitutions for Vegans:

- This recipe is already suitable for vegans.

9. Ginger Peach Iced Tea

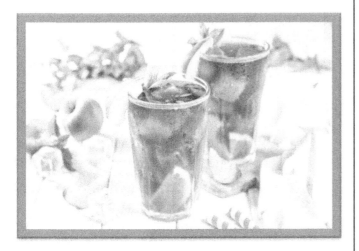

Recipe Description: Ginger Peach Iced Tea is a wonderful choice for seniors, especially during warm weather. This flavorful drink combines ginger's aromatic essence with peaches' sweetness, creating a delightful, diabetic-friendly beverage.

Preparation Time: 10 min (plus chilling time)

Brewing Time: 5 min

Servings: 4

Glycemic Index: Low

Ingredients::

- 4 black tea bags
- 4 cups water
- 1 inch fresh ginger, thinly sliced
- 2 ripe peaches, sliced
- Honey or sugar substitute to taste (optional)
- Ice cubes
- Fresh mint leaves for garnish (optional)

Directions:

1. **Brew the Tea:** Bring water to a boil in a pot or kettle. Remove from heat and add the tea bags. Allow them to steep for about 5 minutes, then remove the tea bags.
2. **Add Ginger and Peaches:** Add the thinly sliced ginger and half of the sliced peaches to the hot tea. Let them infuse for an additional 5 minutes.
3. **Sweeten:** If desired, sweeten with honey or a sugar substitute while the tea is warm. Adjust to your preferred level of sweetness.
4. **Chill:** Allow the tea to cool to room temperature, then refrigerate until cold, which may take 1-2 hours.

5. **Prepare Serving Glasses:** Fill glasses with ice cubes and add peach slices.
6. **Serve:** Strain the tea to remove the ginger and peach slices. Pour the chilled tea over the ice and peach slices in the glasses.
7. **Garnish:** Add a sprig of mint to each glass for a refreshing touch.
8. **Enjoy:** Stir gently and serve the Ginger Peach Iced Tea.

Nutritional Values (per serving):

- Calories: 30 (if honey is added)
- Protein: 0g
- Carbohydrates: 8g (from honey)
- Fat: 0g
- Fiber: 1g
- Sodium: 0mg

Macronutrient Breakdown:

- Protein: 0%
- Carbohydrates: 100% (if honey is added)
- Fat: 0%

Recipe Tips::

- Adjust the amount of ginger based on your preference for spice.
- The tea can be prepared and stored in the refrigerator for 2-3 days.

Allergy Alert::

- No known allergens. Suitable for most dietary needs.

Substitutions for Vegans: Use a vegan-friendly sweetener like agave nectar instead of honey.

10. Raspberry Lemonade

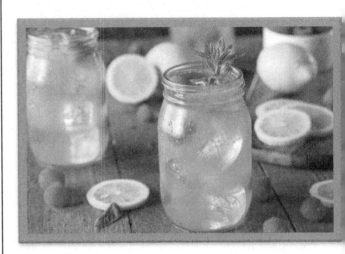

Recipe Description: Raspberry Lemonade is a tangy and delightful beverage, perfect for seniors seeking a refreshing and flavorful drink. This homemade lemonade is enhanced with natural raspberry flavors, making it a diabetic-friendly choice for warm days.

Preparation Time: 10 min

Cooking Time: 0 min

Servings: 4

Glycemic Index: Low

Ingredients::

- 1 cup fresh raspberries
- 1 cup fresh lemon juice (about 4-5 lemons)
- 1/2 cup honey or sugar substitute
- 4 cups water
- Ice cubes
- Additional raspberries and lemon slices for garnish

Directions:

1. **Mash Raspberries:** In a bowl, mash the raspberries to release their juices and flavor.

2. **Make Lemonade Base:** Mix the lemon juice with the honey or sugar substitute in a large pitcher. Stir until the sweetener dissolves completely.

3. **Combine Ingredients::** Add the mashed raspberries to the lemonade base. Mix thoroughly.

4. **Add Water:** Pour water into the pitcher and stir well. Adjust the sweetness or tartness by adding more honey or lemon juice.

5. **Chill:** Refrigerate the lemonade for at least 1 hour to allow the flavors to blend and the drink to chill thoroughly.

6. **Serve:** Fill glasses with ice cubes. Strain the lemonade into the glasses to remove seeds and pulp from the raspberries.

7. **Garnish:** Add a few whole raspberries and a slice of lemon to each glass for an extra touch.

8. **Enjoy:** Serve the raspberry lemonade cold for a refreshing and flavorful drink.

Nutritional Values (per serving):

- Calories: 100 (varies depending on the sweetener used)
- Protein: 1g
- Carbohydrates: 25g
- Fat: 0g
- Fiber: 2g
- Sodium: 5mg

Macronutrient Breakdown:

- Protein: 4%
- Carbohydrates: 96%
- Fat: 0%

Recipe Tips::

- Fresh raspberries provide the best flavor, but frozen raspberries can also be used.
- Adjust the ratio of lemon juice to water depending on how strong or mild you prefer your lemonade.

Allergy Alert::

- No known allergens. Suitable for most dietary needs.

Substitutions for Vegans: This recipe is already vegan-friendly.

GET YOUR BONUSES NOW!

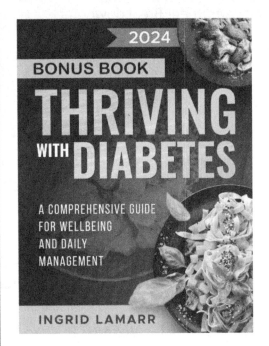
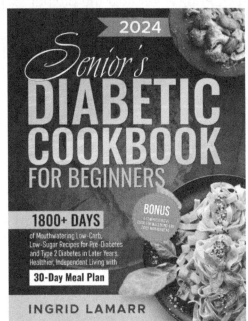

Download your FREE BONUSES now!

https://bit.ly/diabeticlanding

CHAPTER 8: SAUCES AND CONDIMENTS

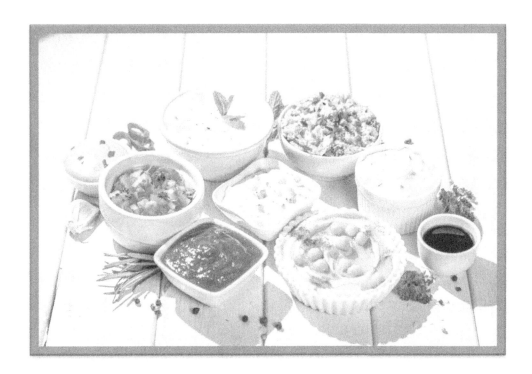

1. Classic Tomato Sauce

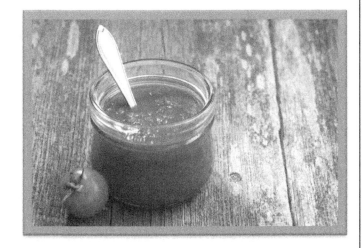

Recipe Description

This diabetic-friendly Classic Tomato Sauce remains a versatile and essential condiment, perfect for seniors. It's simple, flavorful, and suitable for pasta, pizza, and casseroles, with adjustments to reduce sugar content and maintain a low glycemic index.

Preparation Time: 15 min

Cooking Time: 35 min

Servings: 4

Glycemic Index: Low

Ingredients:

- 1 can (28 ounces) crushed tomatoes (no added sugar)
- 1 small onion, finely chopped
- 2 cloves garlic, minced
- 2 tablespoons olive oil
- 1 teaspoon dried basil
- 1 teaspoon dried oregano
- Salt and pepper to taste

- 1 teaspoon erythritol or stevia (optional, instead of sugar)

Directions

1. Sauté Aromatics: Heat olive oil in a saucepan over medium heat. Sauté onion until translucent, about 5-7 minutes. Add minced garlic and cook for 1 minute.
2. Add Tomatoes and Spices: Add crushed tomatoes to the saucepan. Stir in dried basil, oregano, salt, and pepper. Add erythritol or stevia, if using, to balance acidity.
3. Simmer: Bring sauce to a simmer and reduce heat to low. Cook uncovered for about 35 minutes, stirring occasionally.
4. Taste and Adjust: Taste the sauce after simmering. Adjust seasoning or thin with water if needed.
5. Serve or Store: Use immediately or cool and store in an airtight container in the refrigerator for up to a week.

Nutritional Values (per serving)

Calories: 75, Protein: 2g, Carbohydrates: 9g, Fat: 4g, Fiber: 3g, Sodium: 180mg

Macronutrient Breakdown

Protein: 11%, Carbohydrates: 48%, Fat: 41%

Recipe Tips:

- Blend for a smoother sauce if desired.
- Customize with capers, olives, or red pepper flakes for added flavor.

Allergy Alert:

- No major allergens. Suitable for most dietary needs, including diabetes.

Substitutions for Vegans:

This recipe is already vegan-friendly.

2. Honey Mustard Dressing

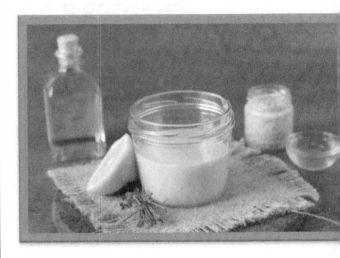

Recipe Description

This diabetic-friendly Honey Mustard Dressing maintains its classic American charm, perfect for seniors. The blend is adjusted for sweetness and tanginess, making it ideal for salads, sandwiches or as a dipping sauce while mindful of blood sugar levels.

Preparation Time: 10 min

Cooking Time: 0 min

Servings: 4 Glycemic Index: Low

Ingredients:

- 1/4 cup sugar-free honey alternative (like stevia-based syrup)
- 1/4 cup Dijon mustard
- 1/4 cup mayonnaise (use egg-free mayonnaise for egg allergies)
- 1 tablespoon apple cider vinegar (for added health benefits)
- Salt and pepper to taste

Directions

1. Combine **Ingredients**:: Mix the sugar-free honey alternative, Dijon mustard,

mayonnaise, and apple cider vinegar until smooth.

2. Season: Adjust flavor with salt and pepper. Add more sweetener for sweetness or more mustard for tanginess.

3. Store or Serve: Use immediately or store in the refrigerator in an airtight container for up to a week.

4. Serve: Drizzle over salads, spread on sandwiches, or use as a dip for snacks.

Nutritional Values (per serving)

Calories: 100, Protein: 0g, Carbohydrates: 10g (from sugar-free sweetener and mustard), Fat: 6g, Fiber: 0g, Sodium: 190mg

Macronutrient Breakdown

Protein: 0%, Carbohydrates: 40%, Fat: 60%

Recipe Tips:

- Substitute Greek yogurt for mayonnaise for a healthier version.
- Adjust consistency with water or more vinegar if desired.

Allergy Alert:

- Contains eggs (if using regular mayonnaise). Use egg-free mayonnaise for egg allergies.

Substitutions for Vegans: Use vegan mayonnaise and a vegan-friendly sweetener like agave syrup.

3. Classic Cranberry Sauce

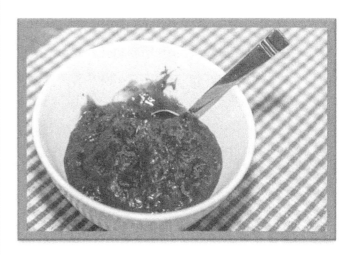

Recipe Description

This diabetic-friendly Classic Cranberry Sauce retains its traditional American charm, perfect for seniors. It offers a simple preparation with a rich, tangy flavor, now adjusted to be more suitable for those managing diabetes, and pairs well with various dishes.

Preparation Time: 10 min

Cooking Time: 20 min

Servings: 4

Glycemic Index: Low

Ingredients:

- 1 cup fresh or frozen cranberries
- 1/2 cup sugar-free orange juice (or water with a squeeze of fresh orange)
- 1/2 cup water
- 1/2 cup erythritol or stevia (adjust quantity based on sweetness level compared to sugar)
- 1 cinnamon stick (optional)
- Zest of one orange (optional)

Directions

1. Combine **Ingredients:**: In a saucepan, mix cranberries, sugar-free orange juice, water, and erythritol or stevia.
2. Add Flavorings: Include a cinnamon stick and orange zest for additional flavor.
3. Cook the Sauce: Bring to a boil over medium-high heat, then simmer.
4. Simmer: Cook for 10-15 minutes, allowing cranberries to burst and thicken the sauce.
5. Stir and Mash: Occasionally stir and mash some cranberries to break them down.
6. Check Consistency: The sauce should thicken according to your preference and will thicken more upon cooling.
7. Cool and Serve: Let cool and remove the cinnamon stick if used.
8. Store or Serve: Serve at room temperature, chilled, or store in the refrigerator for up to a week.

Nutritional Values (per serving)

Calories: 50, Protein: 0g, Carbohydrates: 15g (mostly from cranberries and sugar-free juice), Fat: 0g, Fiber: 2g, Sodium: 0mg

Macronutrient Breakdown

Protein: 0%, Carbohydrates: 100% (natural from cranberries), Fat: 0%

Recipe Tips:
- Adjust sweetness to taste. Add more sweetener for sweetness, or leave it tart.
- Orange juice and zest add a citrusy note but can be omitted for traditional flavor.

Allergy Alert:
- No known allergens. Suitable for most dietary needs, including diabetes.

Substitutions for Vegans:

This recipe is already vegan-friendly.

4. Garlic Herb Butter

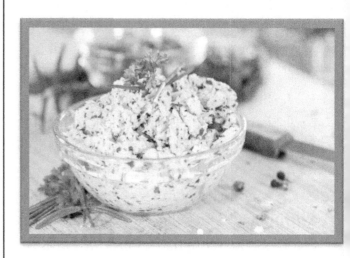

Recipe Description

This diabetic-friendly Garlic Herb Butter, or compound butter, remains a flavorful and versatile condiment, ideal for seniors. It enhances the taste of various dishes, adding rich flavor to vegetables, bread, meats, and more without affecting blood sugar levels.

Preparation Time: 15 min

Cooking Time: 0 min

Servings: 4

Glycemic Index: Low

Ingredients:
- 1/2 cup unsalted butter, softened (or high-quality vegan butter for vegans)
- 3 cloves garlic, minced
- 2 tablespoons fresh parsley, finely chopped
- 1 teaspoon fresh thyme, minced
- 1 teaspoon fresh rosemary, minced
- Salt and pepper to taste

Directions

1. Prepare Butter: Ensure butter is at room temperature for easy mixing. Place in a medium bowl.
2. Add Herbs and Garlic: Mix in minced garlic, parsley, thyme, and rosemary. Fresh herbs are best, but dried herbs can be used (reduce quantity to 1/3).
3. Season: Add salt and pepper to taste.
4. Mix Well: Combine all **Ingredients:** evenly using a fork or hand mixer.
5. Shape Butter: On plastic wrap or parchment paper, wrap butter tightly into a log for easy slicing.
6. Refrigerate: Chill for at least 1 hour to firm up and blend flavors.
7. Serve: Use to top vegetables, spread on bread, or melt over meats.

Nutritional Values (per serving)
Calories: 102, Protein: 0g, Carbohydrates: 1g, Fat: 11g, Fiber: 0g, Sodium: 2mg
Macronutrient Breakdown
Protein: 0%, Carbohydrates: 1%, Fat: 99%

Recipe Tips:
- Adjust herbs and garlic to taste. Add basil or chives for variety.
- Store in the refrigerator for up to 2 weeks or freeze for longer storage.

Allergy Alert:
- Contains dairy. For a dairy-free version, use plant-based butter.

Substitutions for Vegans:
Use a high-quality vegan butter alternative.

5. Avocado Cilantro Lime Dressing

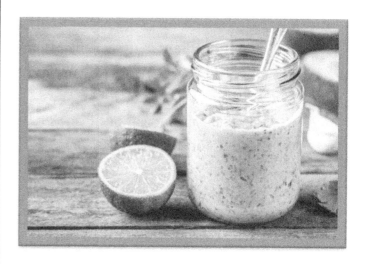

Recipe Description

This diabetic-friendly Avocado Cilantro Lime Dressing offers a creamy, zesty flavor, perfect for seniors who enjoy fresh and vibrant tastes. Ideal as a salad dressing, dip, or sandwich spread, it's made with diabetic-conscious **Ingredients:** to complement a variety of dishes.

Preparation Time: 15 min
Cooking Time: 0 min
Servings: 4
Glycemic Index: Low

Ingredients:
- 1 ripe avocado
- 1/4 cup fresh cilantro, chopped
- Juice of 2 limes
- 1/2 cup Greek yogurt or sour cream (use dairy-free yogurt for a vegan or dairy-free version)
- 2 cloves garlic, minced
- Salt and pepper to taste
- Water for thinning (optional)

Directions

1. Prepare Avocado: Halve the avocado, remove the pit, and scoop the flesh into a blender or food processor.
2. Add **Ingredients:**: Add cilantro, lime juice, Greek yogurt (or sour cream), and garlic to the avocado.
3. Blend: Blend until smooth, adding water if needed for desired consistency.
4. Season: Adjust flavor with salt and pepper.
5. Serve or Store: Use immediately or store in the refrigerator in an airtight container for 2-3 days.
6. Enjoy: Drizzle over salads, use as a vegetable dip, or spread on sandwiches.

Nutritional Values (per serving)

Calories: 85, Protein: 3g, Carbohydrates: 6g, Fat: 7g, Fiber: 4g, Sodium: 30mg

Macronutrient Breakdown

Protein: 14%, Carbohydrates: 28%, Fat: 58%

Recipe Tips:

- Lime juice adds flavor and prevents the browning of avocado.
- Adjust cilantro and garlic to taste.

Allergy Alert:

- Contains dairy. Use dairy-free yogurt for a dairy-free or vegan version.

Substitutions for Vegans:

Replace Greek yogurt with vegan yogurt or blended soaked cashews.

6. Barbecue Sauce

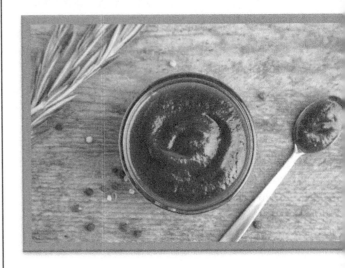

Recipe Description

This diabetic-friendly Barbecue Sauce is an American cuisine staple, suitable for seniors who relish a blend of sweet, tangy, and smoky flavors. It's ideal for grilling, marinating, or as a condiment, modified to suit a diabetic diet while retaining its delicious taste.

Preparation Time: 15 min

Cooking Time: 25 min

Servings: 4

Glycemic Index: Low

Ingredients:

- 1 cup sugar-free ketchup
- 1/4 cup apple cider vinegar
- 1/4 cup erythritol or stevia (instead of brown sugar)
- 1 tablespoon Worcestershire sauce (ensure it's vegan for vegans)
- 1 tablespoon soy sauce (or coconut aminos for soy-free)
- 1 teaspoon smoked paprika
- 1/2 teaspoon garlic powder

- 1/2 teaspoon onion powder
- Salt and pepper to taste
- A dash of hot sauce (optional)

Directions

1. Combine **Ingredients:**: In a saucepan, mix sugar-free ketchup, apple cider vinegar, erythritol or stevia, Worcestershire sauce, soy sauce or coconut aminos, smoked paprika, garlic powder, and onion powder.
2. Simmer: Bring to a simmer over medium heat, stirring to dissolve erythritol or stevia.
3. Season: Adjust seasoning with salt, pepper, and hot sauce if desired.
4. Thicken Sauce: Simmer for 15-20 minutes to desired consistency, stirring occasionally.
5. Cool and Store: Let the sauce cool, then store it in an airtight container in the fridge for up to two weeks.
6. Serve: Use for grilling, marinating, or as a dipping sauce.

Nutritional Values (per serving)

Calories: 60, Protein: 1g, Carbohydrates: 15g (mostly from sugar-free ketchup), Fat: 0g, Fiber: 1g, Sodium: 500mg

Macronutrient Breakdown

Protein: 7%, Carbohydrates: 93%, Fat: 0%

Recipe Tips:

- Add liquid smoke for extra smokiness.
- Vary erythritol or stevia and vinegar for preferred sweetness and tanginess.

Allergy Alert:

- Contains soy. Use coconut aminos for a soy-free version.

Substitutions for Vegans:

Check Worcestershire sauce is vegan; traditional versions contain anchovies. Use coconut aminos instead of soy sauce.

---

7. Lemon Dill Sauce

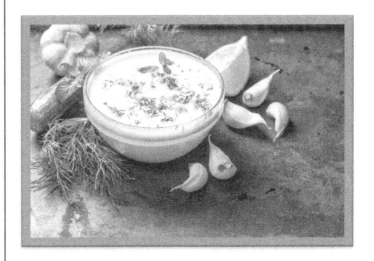

Recipe Description

This diabetic-friendly Lemon Dill Sauce is light and refreshing, perfect for seniors who enjoy citrus and herb flavors. Ideal for complementing fish, chicken, or vegetables, this sauce adds a bright and tangy accent to meals tailored to suit diabetic dietary needs.

Preparation Time: 10 min

Cooking Time: 0 min

Servings: 4

Glycemic Index: Low

Ingredients:

- 1/2 cup Greek yogurt or sour cream (use plant-based yogurt or sour cream for dairy-free and vegan versions)
- 2 tablespoons fresh dill, finely chopped
- Juice of 1 lemon

- 1 teaspoon lemon zest
- 1 clove garlic, minced
- Salt and pepper to taste

Directions

1. Combine Base **Ingredients:**: Mix Greek yogurt (or sour cream) with lemon juice and zest. The lemon provides tanginess and fragrance.
2. Add Herbs and Garlic: Stir in fresh dill and minced garlic. Use dried dill if necessary.
3. Season: Adjust with salt and pepper. Aim for a balanced flavor.
4. Chill (Optional): Refrigerate for an hour for enhanced flavor, or serve immediately.
5. Serve: Drizzle over fish, chicken, or vegetables, or use as a dip or salad dressing.

Nutritional Values (per serving)

Calories: 35, Protein: 3g, Carbohydrates: 4g, Fat: 1g, Fiber: 0g, Sodium: 20mg

Macronutrient Breakdown

Protein: 34%, Carbohydrates: 46%, Fat: 20%

Recipe Tips:

- Modify lemon juice and zest amounts for desired tanginess.
- It can be prepared ahead and refrigerated for up to 3 days.

Allergy Alert:

- Contains dairy. For dairy-free or vegan, use suitable substitutes.

Substitutions for Vegans:

Opt for vegan yogurt or sour cream.

8. Caramelized Onion Relish

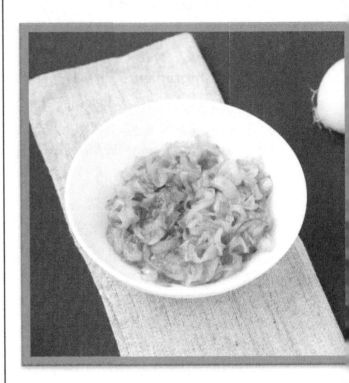

Recipe Description

This diabetic-friendly Caramelized Onion Relish offers a rich blend of sweet and savory flavors, perfect for seniors seeking depth in their condiments. Suitable for serving with meats, sandwiches, or as a topping for grilled vegetables, this version is adjusted to cater to diabetic dietary requirements.

Preparation Time: 15 min

Cooking Time: 35 min

Servings: 4

Glycemic Index: Low

Ingredients:

- 2 large onions, thinly sliced
- 2 tablespoons olive oil
- 1 tablespoon balsamic vinegar

- 1 tablespoon erythritol or stevia (instead of brown sugar)
- Salt and pepper to taste

Directions

1. Caramelize Onions: In a skillet, heat olive oil over medium heat. Add onions and cook for 20-25 minutes until golden brown and soft.
2. Add Flavor: Stir in balsamic vinegar and erythritol or stevia.
3. Season: Adjust the taste with salt and pepper.
4. Reduce: Cook for another 5 minutes, letting flavors combine and mixture thicken slightly.
5. Cool and Serve: Cool and serve warm or at room temperature.
6. Store: Store in an airtight container in the fridge for up to a week.

Nutritional Values (per serving)

Calories: 60, Protein: 1g, Carbohydrates: 7g, Fat: 4g, Fiber: 1g, Sodium: 5mg

Macronutrient Breakdown

Protein: 7%, Carbohydrates: 47%, Fat: 46%

Recipe Tips:

- Slow-cook onions to enhance their natural sweetness.
- Use as a topping for burgers, steaks, or in sandwiches.

Allergy Alert:

- No major allergens. Suitable for most dietary needs.

Substitutions for Vegans:

This recipe is already vegan-friendly.

9. Creamy Horseradish Sauce

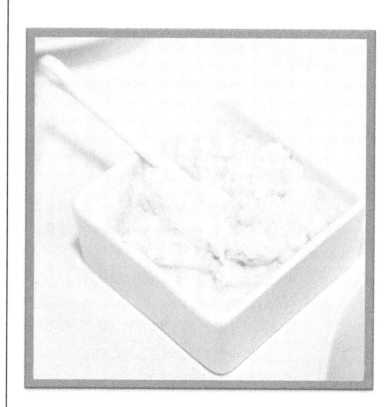

Recipe Description

This diabetic-friendly Creamy Horseradish Sauce is tangy and slightly spicy, ideal for seniors who enjoy bold flavors. It's perfect with roast beef, sandwiches, or as a vegetable dip, made with **Ingredients:** suitable for a diabetic diet.

Preparation Time: 10 min

Cooking Time: 0 min

Servings: 4

Glycemic Index: Low

Ingredients:

- 1/2 cup sour cream (use dairy-free sour cream for vegan and dairy-free versions)
- 2 tablespoons prepared horseradish
- 1 teaspoon Dijon mustard
- 1 teaspoon apple cider vinegar

- 1/2 teaspoon erythritol or stevia (instead of sugar)
- Salt and pepper to taste

Directions

1. Mix Base Ingredients: Combine sour cream, horseradish, and Dijon mustard in a bowl.
2. Add Flavorings: Stir in apple cider vinegar and erythritol or stevia.
3. Season: Adjust with salt and pepper. Modify the horseradish amount for desired spiciness.
4. Combine Thoroughly: Mix well for a smooth texture.
5. Chill (Optional): Refrigerate for about an hour before serving for enhanced flavor, or serve immediately.
6. Serve: Enjoy with roast beef, on sandwiches, or as a dip for veggies.

Nutritional Values (per serving)

Calories: 55, Protein: 1g, Carbohydrates: 3g, Fat: 5g, Fiber: 0g, Sodium: 95mg

Macronutrient Breakdown

Protein: 7%, Carbohydrates: 22%, Fat: 71%

Recipe Tips:

- Control the heat level by adjusting the horseradish.
- Store in an airtight container in the fridge for up to 1 week.

Allergy Alert:

- Contains dairy. Use dairy-free sour cream for dairy-free or vegan needs.

Substitutions for Vegans:

Use a plant-based sour cream alternative.

Inizio modulo

10. Maple Cinnamon Apple Sauce

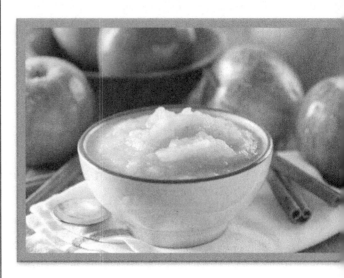

Recipe Description

This diabetic-friendly Maple Cinnamon Apple Sauce is a sweet and comforting condiment for seniors. It's a great accompaniment to breakfast dishes, desserts, or snacks. The flavors of maple and cinnamon are adjusted to suit a diabetic diet while maintaining their delightful depth.

Preparation Time: 15 min

Cooking Time: 25 min

Servings: 4

Glycemic Index: Low

Ingredients:

- 4 large apples, peeled, cored, and chopped (choose varieties with lower natural sugars)
- 1/2 cup water
- 1/4 cup sugar-free maple-flavored syrup (made with sugar substitutes)
- 1/2 teaspoon ground cinnamon
- A pinch of salt

Directions

1. Cook Apples: Combine apples and water in a saucepan. Simmer over medium heat.
2. Simmer: Cover and cook for 15-20 minutes until apples are tender.
3. Add Flavors: Stir in sugar-free maple-flavored syrup, cinnamon, and salt.
4. Mash or Puree: Mash for chunky sauce or blend for a smooth texture.
5. Taste and Adjust: Adjust sweetness or cinnamon to taste.
6. Cool and Serve: Serve warm or chilled.
7. Store: Keep leftovers in an airtight container in the fridge for up to a week.

Nutritional Values (per serving)

Calories: 100, Protein: 0g, Carbohydrates: 25g, Fat: 0g, Fiber: 4g, Sodium: 10mg

Macronutrient Breakdown

Protein: 0%, Carbohydrates: 100% (natural from apples), Fat: 0%

Recipe Tips:
- Select a mix of apple varieties for a balanced flavor.
- Adjust the amount of sugar-free maple syrup to suit your taste.

Allergy Alert:
- No major allergens. Suitable for most dietary needs.

Substitutions for Vegans:

This recipe is already vegan-friendly.

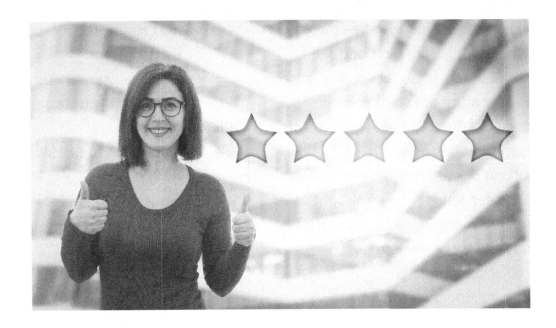

As a publisher, every single review is fundamental support for us. Your voice can make a difference and help us continue our mission. If you believe in the value of what we do and want to lend us a hand, please take a moment to share your thoughts. Your review is our beacon in the vast sea of publishing. From the bottom of our hearts, thank you for your invaluable contribution!

http://bit.ly/diabeticrev

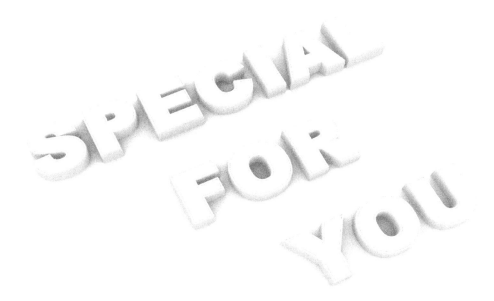

1. Roast Turkey with Herb Butter

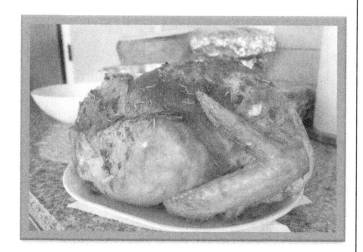

Recipe Description:

This diabetic-friendly version of Roast Turkey with Herb Butter is designed for seniors. It offers a delicious holiday meal option that is moist and flavorful. Combining herbs and butter makes the turkey suitable for those managing diabetes.

Preparation Time: 25 min

Cooking Time: 3 hours (varies based on a 12-pound turkey)

Servings: 6-8

Ingredients::

- 1 whole turkey (12 pounds)
- 1/2 cup unsalted butter, softened
- 2 tablespoons fresh rosemary, chopped
- 2 tablespoons fresh thyme, chopped
- 2 tablespoons fresh sage, chopped
- 2 cloves garlic, minced
- Salt and pepper to taste
- 1 onion, quartered
- 1 lemon, halved

Directions:

1. Preheat the oven to 325°F (165°C).
2. Combine butter, rosemary, thyme, sage, garlic, salt, and pepper to make the herb butter in a bowl.

3. Remove the giblets and neck from the turkey, rinse, and pat dry.

4. Loosen the turkey skin and spread herb butter under the skin and inside the cavity. Apply the remaining butter on the outside.

5. Place onion and lemon in the turkey cavity.

6. Put the turkey breast side up in a roasting pan. Tent with foil to prevent excessive browning.

7. Roast for about 13 minutes per pound, approximately 2 hours, and 36 minutes for a 12-pound turkey.

8. Baste every 45 minutes with pan juices.

9. When the thigh's internal temperature reaches 165°F (74°C), Turkey is done.

10. Let the turkey rest for 20 minutes before carving.

Nutritional Values (per serving):

- Calories: Approximately 450-550
- Protein: ~70g
- Carbohydrates: ~1g
- Fat: ~20g
- Fiber: 0g
- Sodium: ~200mg

Recipe Tips::

- Adjust herbs to taste.
- Resting the turkey is crucial for juicy meat.

Allergy Alert:: Contains dairy (butter).

Substitutions for Vegans: This recipe is not applicable as it involves a whole turkey. Consider a plant-based roast for a vegan alternative.

2. Green Bean Casserole

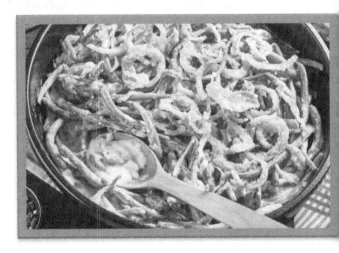

Recipe Description: A healthier twist on the classic Green Bean Casserole, perfect for seniors managing diabetes. This version uses low-fat and sugar-free **Ingredients:** while maintaining the comforting and creamy flavors of the original dish.

Preparation Time: 15 min

Cooking Time: 30 min

Servings: 6

Glycemic Index: Low to Medium

Ingredients::

- 1 lb fresh green beans, trimmed and cut into bite-sized pieces
- 1 can (10.5 oz) of low-fat, no added sugar cream of mushroom soup
- 1/2 cup skim milk
- 1 teaspoon low-sodium soy sauce
- 1/4 teaspoon black pepper
- 1 1/2 cups crispy fried onions (look for lower-sodium, no sugar added variety)

Directions:

1. **Preheat Oven & Prepare Beans:** Prehea your oven to 350°F (175°C). Boil a pot of water and blanch the green beans for

about 5 minutes until tender. Drain and set aside.

2. **Mix Sauce Ingredients::** In a large bowl, mix the low-fat cream of mushroom soup, skim milk, soy sauce, and black pepper to create a lighter, creamy sauce.

3. **Combine Beans with Sauce:** Add the blanched green beans to the bowl with the sauce. Toss gently to ensure the beans are evenly coated.

4. **Assemble Casserole:** Transfer the green bean mixture to a greased baking dish. Spread out evenly.

5. **Add Fried Onions:** Sprinkle half of the crispy fried onions over the top of the green bean mixture.

6. **Bake** in the oven for about 25 minutes until the mixture is hot and bubbling.

7. **Add More Onions & Final Bake:** Remove the casserole from the oven. Sprinkle the remaining fried onions and bake for 5 minutes, until the onions are golden brown.

8. **Serve:** Let the casserole cool for a few minutes before serving. It's best enjoyed warm.

Nutritional Values (approx. per serving):
- Calories: 160
- Protein: 4g
- Carbohydrates: 14g
- Fat: 10g
- Fiber: 2g
- Sodium: 450mg

Recipe Tips::
- Opt for fresh green beans for the best texture and nutritional value.

- If you prefer, use low-fat yogurt instead of cream of mushroom soup for a different version.
- Adjust seasonings to taste.

Allergy Alert::
- Contains dairy and soy. Check the **Ingredients:** in the fried onions for potential allergens.

Substitutions for Vegans:
- Replace the cream of mushroom soup with a vegan alternative.
- Use almond milk or another plant-based milk instead of dairy milk.
- Opt for vegan-friendly crispy fried onions.

3. Classic Mashed Potatoes

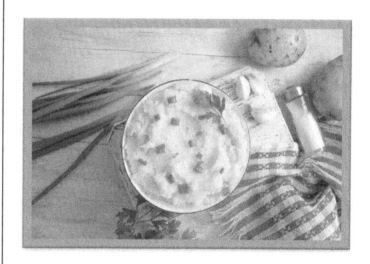

Recipe Description

Classic Mashed Potatoes are a staple in American holiday meals, loved by seniors for their creamy texture and comforting taste. This simple recipe brings out the best in potatoes with butter and milk.

Preparation Time: 15 min

Cooking Time: 20 min

Servings: 6

Glycemic Index: Medium

Ingredients:

- 2 lbs Yukon Gold or Russet potatoes, peeled and quartered
- 1/2 cup milk
- 1/4 cup unsalted butter
- Salt and pepper to taste

Directions

1. **Boil Potatoes:** Place the peeled and quartered potatoes in a large pot and cover them with cold water. Bring to a boil over high heat, then reduce to a simmer. Cook until the potatoes are tender, about 15-20 minutes.

2. **Heat Milk and Butter:** While the potatoes are cooking, heat the milk and butter in a small saucepan or microwave until the butter is melted and the milk is warm.

3. **Drain and Mash Potatoes:** Once the potatoes are cooked, drain them well and return them to the pot. Use a potato masher to mash them to your desired consistency.

4. **Add Milk and Butter:** Gradually add the warm milk and butter mixture to the potatoes, stirring and mashing until they are creamy and smooth.

5. **Season:** Add salt and pepper to taste. Continue to mash and mix until everything is well combined, and the potatoes are fluffy.

6. **Serve:** Serve the mashed potatoes warm. They are perfect with gravy, roast meats, or alone.

Nutritional Values (per serving)

Calories: 200, Protein: 4g, Carbohydrates: 30g, Fat: 8g, Fiber: 2g, Sodium: 20mg

Macronutrient Breakdown

Protein: 8%, Carbohydrates: 60%, Fat: 32%

Recipe Tips:

- For extra creamy potatoes, you can use cream instead of milk.
- For a lighter version, use low-fat milk and less butter.

Allergy Alert:

- Contains dairy. For a dairy-free version, use plant-based milk and butter substitutes.

Substitutions for Vegans: Use a vegan butter substitute and plant-based milk.

---

4. Sweet Potato Casserole with Low-Glycemic Topping

Preparation Time: 15 min

Cooking Time: 30 min

Servings: 6

Glycemic Index: Medium

Ingredients:

- 4 large sweet potatoes, peeled and cut into chunks
- 1/4 cup unsalted butter, melted
- 1/3 cup milk (preferably almond or another low-glycemic alternative)
- 1/4 cup erythritol or another sugar substitute
- 1 teaspoon vanilla extract
- 1/2 teaspoon cinnamon
- 1/4 teaspoon nutmeg
- Salt to taste
- 2 cups chopped nuts (like pecans or walnuts) for topping

Directions

1. **Cook Sweet Potatoes:** Boil sweet potato chunks until tender (15-20 minutes). Drain well.
2. **Mash and Mix:** Mash sweet potatoes with melted butter, milk, sugar substitute, vanilla, cinnamon, nutmeg, and salt.
3. **Preheat Oven:** Set to 350°F (175°C).
4. **Prepare Casserole:** Spread the sweet potato mixture into a greased baking dish.
5. **Add Topping:** Sprinkle chopped nuts over the sweet potato mixture.
6. **Bake:** For 15-20 minutes or until the topping is lightly browned.
7. **Cool and Serve:** Let it cool slightly before serving.

Nutritional Values (approximation per serving)

- Calories: 250
- Protein: 4g
- Carbohydrates: 35g (complex, from sweet potatoes)
- Fat: 12g (mostly from nuts)
- Fiber: 5g
- Sodium: 70mg

Recipe Tips:

- Substitute sugar with erythritol to reduce the glycemic load.
- Nuts add a crunchy texture and are a healthier alternative to marshmallows.
- Adjust spices to taste.

Allergy Alert:

- Contains dairy. Use dairy-free milk and butter substitutes for dairy allergies.

Substitutions for Vegans

- Replace butter with vegan butter.
- Use plant-based milk.

5. Traditional Pumpkin Pie

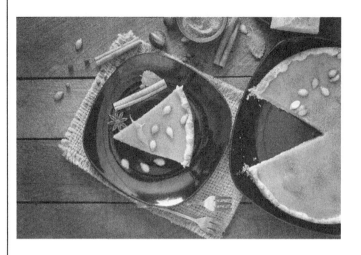

Preparation Time: 20 min

Cooking Time: 55 min

Servings: 8

Glycemic Index: Medium

Ingredients:

- 1 (9-inch) unbaked pie crust (whole wheat or gluten-free, if needed)
- 1 can (15 oz) pumpkin puree
- 3/4 cup erythritol or another suitable sugar substitute
- 1/2 cup unsweetened almond milk
- 1/2 cup heavy cream (or coconut cream for a dairy-free version)
- 2 eggs (or vegan egg substitute)
- 1 teaspoon ground cinnamon
- 1/2 teaspoon ground ginger
- 1/4 teaspoon ground nutmeg
- 1/4 teaspoon ground cloves
- 1/2 teaspoon salt

Directions

1. **Preheat Oven:** To 425°F (220°C).
2. **Prepare Filling:** Mix pumpkin puree, sugar substitute, almond milk, cream, and eggs. Add cinnamon, ginger, nutmeg, cloves, and salt.

3. **Fill Pie Crust:** Pour mixture into unbaked pie crust.
4. **Bake:** Bake for 15 minutes at 425°F, then reduce heat to 350°F (175 °C) and bake for 40 more minutes or until set.
5. **Cool:** Allow to cool on a wire rack.
6. **Serve:** Enjoy at room temperature or chilled.

Nutritional Values (approximation per serving)

- Calories: 280
- Protein: 4g
- Carbohydrates: 30g (complex, lower impact due to sugar substitute)
- Fat: 15g
- Fiber: 3g
- Sodium: 200mg

Recipe Tips:

- Sugar substitute like erythritol reduces glycemic impact.
- Use almond milk and coconut cream for a lower-fat and dairy-free option.
- Vegan egg substitutes are available for a vegan diet.

Allergy Alert:

- Contains eggs and dairy (if using traditional **Ingredients:**).
- Contains gluten (if using a regular pie crust).

Substitutions for Vegans

- Use a vegan pie crust, plant-based milk, coconut cream, and vegan egg replacer.

6. Glazed Ham with Pineapple and Cherries

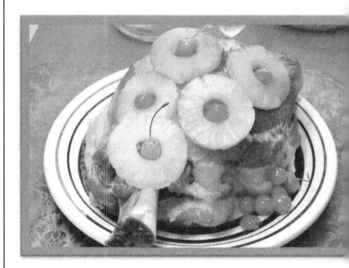

Preparation Time: 20 min

Cooking Time: 1 hour 30 min

Servings: 8-10

Glycemic Index: Low to Medium

Ingredients:

- 1 bone-in fully cooked ham (about 8-10 pounds, low-sodium version)
- 20 oz can pineapple slices in juice, no added sugar
- 10 maraschino cherries, sugar-free if available
- 1 cup erythritol or stevia blend (instead o brown sugar)
- 2 tablespoons Dijon mustard
- 1 tablespoon apple cider vinegar

Directions

1. **Preheat Oven:** To 325°F (163°C).
2. **Prepare Ham:** Place in a roasting pan. Score the surface.
3. **Make Glaze:** Combine erythritol or stevi mustard, vinegar, and half of the

pineapple juice. Heat until the sweetener dissolves.

4. **Glaze Ham:** Brush a third of the glaze on the ham.

5. **Bake:** For 1 hour 30 minutes, basting every 30 minutes with glaze.

6. **Add Pineapple and Cherries:** In the last 30 minutes, decorate the ham with pineapple slices and cherries.

7. **Finish Baking:** Until heated through and glazed.

8. **Rest and Serve:** Rest for 10 minutes before slicing.

Nutritional Values (approximation per serving)

- Calories: 350
- Protein: 40g
- Carbohydrates: 15g (lower due to sugar substitute)
- Fat: 12g
- Fiber: 1g
- Sodium: 1200mg (reduced by using low-sodium ham)

Recipe Tips:

- Use low-sodium ham to reduce overall sodium content.
- Sugar substitutes like erythritol minimize glycemic impact.
- Pineapple and cherries should be in juice, not syrup, and sugar-free if possible.

Allergy Alert:

- No major allergens.

Substitutions for Vegans

- It is not applicable as the main ingredient is ham. Consider a plant-based ham substitute for a vegan alternative, adjusting cooking times as needed.

7. Herb-Roasted Root Vegetables

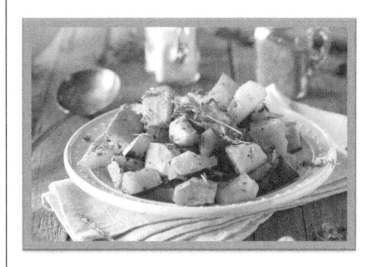

Recipe Description

Herb-Roasted Root Vegetables are a healthy and flavorful side dish, perfect for holiday meals. This dish is ideal for seniors, offering a mix of nutrient-rich vegetables with a rustic and comforting flavor.

Preparation Time: 15 min

Cooking Time: 40 min

Servings: 6

Glycemic Index: Low

Ingredients:

- 2 carrots, peeled and cut into chunks
- 2 parsnips, peeled and cut into chunks
- 1 sweet potato, peeled and cut into chunks
- 1 turnip, peeled and cut into chunks
- 1 red onion, cut into wedges
- 2 tablespoons olive oil
- 1 teaspoon dried rosemary
- 1 teaspoon dried thyme
- Salt and pepper to taste

Directions

1. **Preheat Oven:** Preheat your oven to 400°F (200°C).

2. **Prepare Vegetables:** Peel and cut the carrots, parsnips, sweet potato, and turnip into roughly equal-sized chunks. Cut the red onion into wedges.

3. **Season:** In a large bowl, toss the vegetables with olive oil, dried rosemary, dried thyme, salt, and pepper. Ensure all the vegetables are evenly coated with the oil and herbs.

4. **Roast:** Spread the vegetables in a single layer on a baking sheet. Roast in the oven for about 40 minutes, or until the vegetables are tender and caramelized, stirring halfway through the cooking time.

5. **Serve:** Remove the vegetables from the oven and transfer them to a serving dish. They can be served hot or at room temperature.

Nutritional Values (per serving)

Calories: 140, Protein: 2g, Carbohydrates: 20g, Fat: 7g, Fiber: 4g, Sodium: 40mg

Macronutrient Breakdown

Protein: 6%, Carbohydrates: 57%, Fat: 37%

Recipe Tips:

- You can use any combination of root vegetables you prefer or have on hand.
- Add a splash of balsamic vinegar for an extra flavor boost before serving.

Allergy Alert:

- No major allergens. Suitable for most dietary needs.

Substitutions for Vegans: This recipe is already vegan-friendly.

8. Cranberry Orange Relish

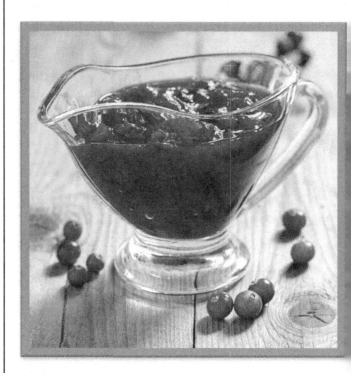

Recipe Description

Cranberry Orange Relish is a vibrant and fresh side dish, perfect for holiday gatherings. This no-cook recipe is especially popular among seniors for its tangy and sweet flavors, and it pairs beautifully with turkey or other holiday meats.

Preparation Time: 10 min

Cooking Time: 0 min

Servings: 6

Glycemic Index: Low

Ingredients:

- 12 oz fresh cranberries
- 1 large orange, zest, and fruit
- 1/2 cup sugar or sugar substitute
- 1/2 teaspoon ground cinnamon
- 1/4 teaspoon ground nutmeg

Directions

1. **Prepare Ingredients::** Wash the cranberries and discard any soft or

bruised ones. Zest the orange and peel it, removing as much white pith as possible.

2. **Blend Cranberries and Orange:** Combine the cranberries and orange segments (with zest) in a food processor. Pulse until the mixture is coarsely chopped but not pureed.

3. **Add Sweeteners and Spices:** Transfer the chopped cranberries and orange to a bowl. Stir in the sugar (or sugar substitute), cinnamon, and nutmeg. Mix well.

4. **Let It Sit:** Allow the relish to sit at room temperature for at least 30 minutes before serving. This resting period lets the flavors meld together.

5. **Serve:** Serve the cranberry orange relish as a condiment with your holiday meal. It's particularly delicious with roast turkey or ham.

Nutritional Values (per serving)

Calories: 90, Protein: 0g, Carbohydrates: 23g, Fat: 0g, Fiber: 2g, Sodium: 0mg

Macronutrient Breakdown

Protein: 0%, Carbohydrates: 100%, Fat: 0%

Recipe Tips:

- Adjust the amount of sugar based on your sweetness preference and the tartness of the cranberries.
- The relish can be made a day in advance and stored in the refrigerator.

Allergy Alert:

- No major allergens. Suitable for most dietary needs.

Substitutions for Vegans: This recipe is already vegan-friendly.

9. Baked Brie and Almonds

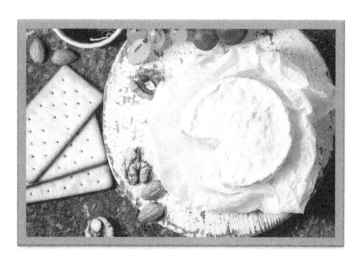

Recipe Description:

A luxurious yet simple appetizer, Baked Brie with Low-Glycemic Sweetener and Almonds is perfect for special occasions. This version is adapted for seniors managing diabetes, offering a creamy texture with a sweet and nutty topping without the high sugar content of traditional recipes.

Preparation Time: 5 minutes

Cooking Time: 15 minutes

Servings: 6

Glycemic Index: Low

Ingredients::

- 1 whole brie cheese (about 8 ounces)
- 2 tablespoons of a low-glycemic sweetener like stevia-based syrup or agave nectar
- 1/4 cup sliced almonds
- Vegetable sticks or low-carb crackers for serving

Directions:

1. **Preheat the Oven:** Set your oven to 350°F (175°C).

2. **Prepare the Brie:** Place the brie on a baking sheet lined with parchment paper. Keep the rind on as it's edible and helps hold the cheese together while baking.

3. **Add Toppings:** Drizzle the low-glycemic sweetener over the brie. Evenly sprinkle the sliced almonds over the top.

4. **Bake:** Bake in the oven for about 15 minutes, or until the cheese is slightly gooey inside and the almonds are lightly toasted.

5. **Serve:** Carefully transfer the baked brie to a serving platter. Serve warm with vegetable sticks or low-carb crackers for a diabetic-friendly option.

Nutritional Values (per serving):

- Calories: 170
- Protein: 8g
- Carbohydrates: 7g
- Fat: 13g
- Fiber: 1g
- Sodium: 180mg

Macronutrient Breakdown:

- Protein: 19%
- Carbohydrates: 16%
- Fat: 65%

Recipe Tips::

- Watch the brie closely while it bakes to ensure it doesn't over-melt.
- Add a sprinkle of fresh thyme or rosemary for an extra flavor dimension before baking.

Allergy Alert::

Contains dairy and nuts. For a nut-free version, omit the almonds.

Substitutions for Vegans:

Use a vegan brie-style cheese and ensure the sweetener is vegan-friendly.

10. Eggnog

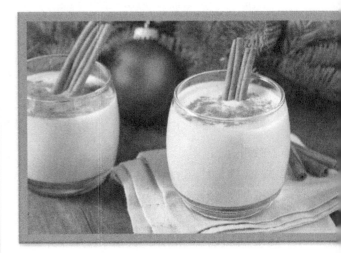

Recipe Description:

Eggnog, a traditional holiday beverage in the United States, is beloved for its rich, creamy texture and festive flavor. This homemade version is modified to be diabetic-friendly, using low-glycemic sweeteners, making it a delightful treat for seniors during special occasions.

Preparation Time: 10 minutes

Cooking Time: 10 minutes (plus chilling time)

Servings: 6

Glycemic Index: Medium

Ingredients::

- 4 cups low-fat milk or plant-based milk
- 1/2 cup low-glycemic sweetener like stevia or erythritol
- 6 large egg yolks
- 1/2 teaspoon ground nutmeg
- 1 teaspoon vanilla extract
- 1/2 cup light cream or dairy-free cream alternative (optional, for a richer eggnog

- Whiskey, brandy, or rum (optional for an adult version)

Directions:

1. **Heat Milk:** Gently warm the milk in a large saucepan over medium-low heat until it's warm but not boiling.
2. **Whisk Egg Yolks and Sweetener:** Whisk the egg yolks with the sweetener in a separate bowl until the mixture is pale and thick.
3. **Temper Egg Mixture:** Gradually add the warm milk to the egg yolk mixture, whisking constantly to prevent the eggs from cooking.
4. **Cook Eggnog:** Return the mixture to the saucepan and cook over low heat, stirring constantly, until it thickens enough to coat the back of a spoon.
5. **Add Flavors:** Remove from heat and stir in ground nutmeg and vanilla extract. If using, add the light cream for a richer texture.
6. **Chill:** Transfer the eggnog to a pitcher or bowl, cover, and chill in the refrigerator for at least an hour.
7. **Serve:** Serve chilled. Add a splash of whiskey, brandy, or rum to each glass if desired. Garnish with a sprinkle of nutmeg or cinnamon.

Nutritional Values (per serving):

- Calories: 220
- Protein: 8g
- Carbohydrates: 20g
- Fat: 12g
- Fiber: 0g
- Sodium: 70mg

Macronutrient Breakdown:

- Protein: 15%
- Carbohydrates: 36%
- Fat: 49%

Recipe Tips::

- For a lighter version, use 2% milk instead of whole milk and reduce or omit the heavy cream.
- Ensure the eggnog doesn't boil during cooking to avoid curdling.

Allergy Alert:: Contains dairy and eggs. For a dairy-free version, use plant-based milk and a vegan egg substitute.

Substitutions for Vegans: Use plant-bas

CHAPTER 10: PRACTICAL TIPS IN THE KITCHEN

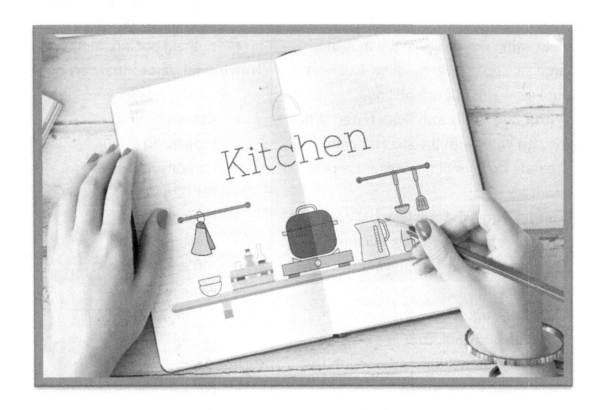

COOKING TECHNIQUES: INTRODUCTION TO HEALTHY COOKING TECHNIQUES.

Eating profoundly affects our emotions, and eating a balanced diet maintains our bodies and minds functioning at their peak. Most of us already know the fundamentals of a healthy diet: stick to the food pyramid, prioritize whole foods, and consume more sugar, salt, and oil.

You start with the greatest **Ingredients:** because you are concerned about your health. Whole grains, organic veggies grown nearby, and fresh, free-range eggs directly from the farmer's market are all staples in your home. But cooking methods are equally as crucial as **Ingredients:**.

- **Braising**: Braising is a combination of sauteing and slow cooking. The meal should be cooked gently in a covered dish after being sautéed over high heat until it is browned on all sides. Most braising recipes need extra liquid; however, you might wish to try wet and dry braising.

- **Broiling**: Food is cooked directly over a high heat source when broiling. This technique swiftly cooks various foods, including vegetables, skinless chicken breasts, and pork chops. Additionally, it's a particularly healthful method of cooking high-fat meats like fish or beef.

Most broilers have a broiling rack and pan underneath a heat source, which can be either an open flame or a heating element; however, the layout can vary based on the oven. This technique resembles grilling in reverse. Like grilling, broiling eliminates saturated fats and gives you a perfectly crisp outside without using any oil. However, the rendered fat gathers in the broiling pan for convenient disposal rather than dripping into an open grill.

- **Roasting**: Similar to broiling and dry braising, roasting is a method that employs low heat to help retain the vitamins and other nutrients in food.

Using high temperatures, hot, dry air is emitted around the meal during roasting. Although the most popular type is an oven, consider any technology that creates a comparable environment. If your oven is otherwise busy, consider a stovetop roaster made of stainless steel. A backyard fire pit will also produce a hot, dry atmosphere for spit roasting.

- **Stir-Fry**: It might surprise you that stir-frying is among the healthiest cooking techniques. After all, you're already aware of the advantages of an oil-free diet, and most versions served in restaurants begin with oil. Stir-frying has historically used very high heat, which might deplete important nutrients.

MEAL PREPARATION: TIPS ON HOW TO PLAN AND PREPARE MEALS FOR THE WEEK

Having well-planned meals and snacks can support you through hectic times. Meal planning helps cut down on food waste and is efficient. Just make sure you follow your shopping list.

- **Thoroughly plan**: ensure you set aside time weekly to plan a meal. Consider the number of meals you would have to prepare for the week and when you need to make quick meals and make them in advance.
- **Check what you have**: Examine your current **Ingredients:** in your pantry, refrigerator, or freezer. Plan your meals around the items you need to use up by looking up their "use-by" dates. The way you keep food has a huge impact on how long it lasts. Take note of the following;
  - Check the label for advice on how to keep food.
  - Place new items at the back and older items at the front of the fridge/ cupboard.
  - Label all foods with the name and the date before you freeze them so they can be easily identified.
- Add some of your favorite meals;
  - Create your favorite go-to list of meals.
  - Introduce new recipes when you have extra time.
  - Consider a themed night, like Meatless Monday, for instance.
- Use up your leftovers.
  - Plan meals like pasta bakes, soups, shepherd's pies, lasagnas, curries, or beef stews that can be chilled and reheated or served cold the following day.
  - Toss leftover meat into a curry or stir-fry, or use leftover veggies in an omelet, soup, or salad.

- ○ Remember that food in the refrigerator must be consumed within three days.
- Cook in bulk
  - ○ Make extra and keep it in the fridge or freezer for later use. Pies, stews, casseroles, and curries all store nicely.
  - ○ Consider what else you may prepare in parallel if you are using the oven. You may prepare some chicken breasts for sandwiches if you're making a casserole.
- Make **Ingredients:** work
  - ○ Select recipes like roast chicken, stir-fried chicken, and chicken sandwiches that all employ the same essential components.
  - ○ Add one or two primary vegetables to a dish, including meat, pasta, or seafood. For instance, you may stir-fry beef with peppers, broccoli, and sweetcorn, or you can use them to make a vegetable pasta bake and serve them with fish or pork.

KITCHEN ORGANIZATION: SUGGESTIONS FOR EFFECTIVELY ORGANIZING THE KITCHEN AND UTENSILS.

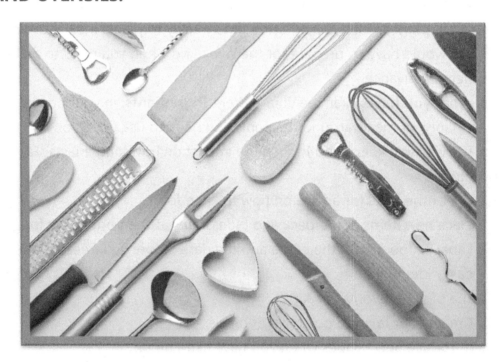

Thanks to these kitchen utensil organizing ideas, you won't have to battle to keep your utensils nea Over time, one can accumulate an immense variety of kitchenware. Some are meant for specialized uses that you might need only once a year, while others are used daily. Using these clever solutions for arranging kitchen utensils, you can cook with greater convenience and less clutter on your counter.

- **Declutter**: Decluttering thoroughly is the first step in every organization's effort, and organizing kitchen utensils is no exception. Ensure your kitchen drawers are free of items you don't use. Be sincere and only save items you will use today, not those you may use in the future or those you have previously used.
- **Separate into categories**: Organizing your commonly used utensils into a drawer is the easiest solution. To keep utensils nice and neat in the drawer, you may easily pick up expandable drawer dividers and trays for organizing utensils. The kitchen will look more orderly if the utensils are stored away from the countertop. If everything you need must be available, store necessities in a drawer close to where you need them.
- Identify frequent-use and seldom-use kitchen utensils.
- Put utensils in drawers close to where they will be used.
- Put in a utensil holder on the counter.
- Repurpose pitchers or vases you already have.
- **Use vertical wall space:** Kitchen utensils can be hung on the wall in several ways. You can use magnetic wall-mounted bars, cup hooks, Command hooks (even elegant silver ones that don't look like regular Command hooks), and bars that carry culinary utensils.

A big kitchen pegboard is useful if you are searching for a more distinctive way to store your utensils. Use hooks to hold the utensils and put them on a nearby wall or over the stove. Pegboard is surprisingly inexpensive, and your neighborhood hardware store will happily cut it to the exact size you want for free.

- Make use of the sides of the upper and lower kitchen cabinets.
- Make use of the inside of cabinet doors.
- Use the side walls inside the pantry.

CHAPTER 11: MANAGING DIABETES IN THE LONG TERM

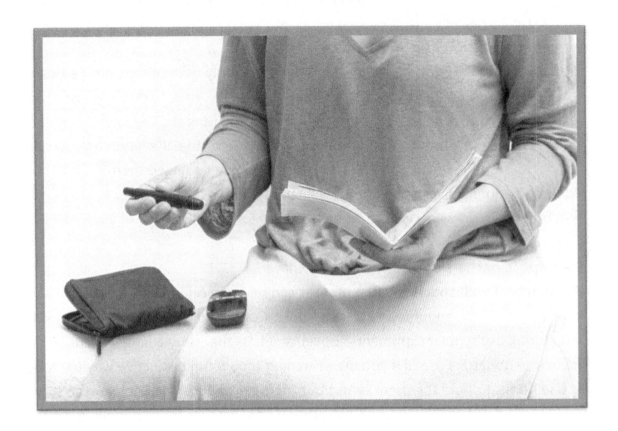

LIFESTYLE AND DIABETES: TIPS ON PHYSICAL EXERCISE, STRESS MANAGEMENT, AND GENERAL LIFESTYLE FOR MANAGING DIABETES.

Maintaining your blood sugar levels within your doctor has prescribed range can be difficult. This is because various unpredictable factors can alter your blood sugar levels. The factors listed below may have an impact on your blood sugar levels.

Food

Whether diabetic or not, a good diet is the foundation of a healthy lifestyle. However, being diabetic means you should be aware of how diet affects blood sugar levels. It's not just about what kind of food you consume; it's also about how much and how you combine different meal kinds.

- **Learn about carbohydrate counting and portion size**: A key to many diabetes management plans is learning carb counting. Carbs, most of the time, highly affect blood sugar levels. Knowing the total carbohydrates they consume for the correct insulin dose is important for those taking mealtime insulin.

- **Consume a balanced diet**: Make a plan for each meal to have a good mix of starch, fruits, vegetables, proteins, and fats. Also, pay attention to the type of carbohydrate you choose. Certain carbs, such as those in fruits, vegetables, and whole grains, are healthier than others. These foods contain fiber, which helps stabilize blood sugar levels, and are low in carbohydrates. Consult a doctor, nurse, or nutritionist for advice on the best foods to eat and how to balance different meal kinds.

- **Avoid sugar-sweetened beverages**: Beverages with added sugar usually have minimal nutritional value and are heavy in calories. Additionally, diabetic individuals should stay away from these drinks because they quickly increase blood sugar levels.

The only exception is if your blood sugar is low. Drinks with added sugar, like soda, juice, and sports drinks, can be a useful remedy for rapidly boosting hypoglycemic blood sugar.

Exercise

Another crucial component of your diabetes control strategy is physical activity. Your muscles use glucose, or sugar, as energy while you work out. Frequent exercise also improves the body's ability to utilize insulin.

Together, these elements lessen your blood sugar levels. The higher the duration of the effect, the more intense your workout. However, even simple tasks like cleaning, gardening, or standing for extended time can lower blood sugar.

- **Talk to your doctor about an exercise plan**: Find out what exercise is right for you. Most adults should engage in moderate aerobic activity for at least one hundred and fifty minutes weekly. On most days of the week, try to get in around thirty minutes of moderate aerobic exercise daily.

Your doctor might first want to assess your general health before making any recommendations if you haven't been active. They can provide an appropriate mix of cardio and muscle-building exercises.

- **Keep an exercise schedule and know your numbers**: Discuss with your physician the ideal time to work out so that it doesn't conflict with your eating and medication schedules. Consult your physician before starting an exercise regimen to determine your ideal blood sugar levels.
- **Remain hydrated**: drinking lots of water or other fluids while exercising due to hydration can influence blood sugar levels.

- **Be prepared**: Try to get some snacks to keep your stomach full and give you energy during an exercise. You can also take some glucose tablets to protect you from low blood sugar levels. Since exercise can harm your health, try to wear a medical identification bracelet to know your blood sugar level.

Medication

When diet and exercise are insufficient to manage your diabetes, insulin, and other diabetes treatments work to lower your blood sugar levels. However, the time and dosage of these drugs determine how effective they are. You may also have changes in your blood sugar levels from medications you use for ailments other than diabetes.

- Store insulin properly: insulin that is improperly stored or has passed its expiration date may not be effective. Insulin is especially sensitive to extremes in temperature.
- Be cautious with new medications: Ask your doctor or pharmacist whether a medicine may influence your blood sugar levels if you're considering taking an over-the-counter medication or if your doctor has prescribed a new prescription to address a different problem, such as high blood pressure or high cholesterol. Sometimes, a different drug might be suggested. Before starting any new over-the-counter medicine, consult your doctor so you are aware of any potential effects on your blood sugar.

Stress

Your blood sugar level may increase if you're under a lot of stress because of the hormones your body releases as a reaction. Furthermore, if you're experiencing a lot of additional stress, it could be more difficult to adhere to your regular diabetes treatment regimen.

- **Look for patterns:** log your stress on a scale of 1 to 10 each time you log your blood sugar level. You'll start noticing a pattern.
- **Take control**: After being aware of stress's impact on your blood sugar, take action. Establish boundaries, decide which task is more important, and learn relaxing techniques. Remain away from typical stressors whenever you can. Exercise frequently aids in blood sugar regulation and stress relief.
- **Get help**: Discover fresh coping mechanisms for stress. Working with a psychologist or clinical social worker can assist you in recognizing pressures, resolving difficult issues, or acquiring new coping mechanisms.

Menstruation and menopause (For the ladies)

As hormone levels change, blood sugar levels might fluctuate significantly during the week before and during menstruation.

Things to do:

- **Search for patterns**: Ensure you monitor your monthly blood sugar readings to predict changes associated with your menstrual cycle.
- **Adjust your diabetes treatment plan as required**: Listen and heed your healthcare provider's advice concerning your meal plan, exercise, or diabetes drugs to manage blood sugar changes.
- **Check blood sugar more frequently**: Ask your doctor if you should monitor your blood sugar more frequently if you are possibly nearing or mid-menopause. Menopause symptoms can occasionally be mistaken for low blood sugar symptoms. Before treating a suspected low take a blood sugar reading to confirm the low blood sugar level.

CHAPTER 12: RESOURCES AND SUPPORT

WHERE TO FIND HELP: RESOURCES AND INFORMATION ON WHERE TO FIND SUPPORT AND ADDITIONAL INFORMATION.

American Diabetes Care and Education Specialists (ADCES) Meeting

The editors of Everyday Health go to the ADCES annual meeting to network with registered dietitians, certified diabetes care and education specialists, and individuals like you who want to improve blood sugar, medicine, food, and other aspects of their lives. You can always check online for information regarding their next meeting.

American Diabetes Association (ADA)

For information on type 1 and type 2 diabetes, the American Diabetes Association is regarded as the top NGO. For those new to living with diabetes, the American Diabetes Association's free annual program, Living With Diabetes, provides excellent resources. Among other benefits, you'll have access to their professional Q&A session, online support system, and newsletter.

American Heart Association (AHA)

AHA's Know Diabetes by Heart is a great resource for heart disease prevention. The ADA-backed program provides comprehensive instruction on maintaining heart health while managing diabetes.

Cleveland Clinic Functional Ketogenic Program

Have you considered trying the ketogenic (or "keto") diet for improved diabetes management? This ground-breaking Cleveland Clinic program provides a means to achieve precisely that, with qualified counselors available to modify your medicine and diet.

Diabetes Daily

You won't feel as alone in your diabetes journey after visiting this website. In addition to their forum, where you may connect with other people managing diabetes, they have a ton of inspirational patient tales.

Diabetes Sisters

These sisters genuinely care about you regarding administering insulin at mealtimes, prioritizing your mental well-being, and any other issues you may not know how to discuss with your diabetes care team. Every three to six months, they switch up the bloggers who share their accounts of living with diabetes. Furthermore, despite the website's name, "Diabetes Misters" are also invited.

Conclusion: Embracing a Healthier Future

As we reach the end of our journey together through "Senior's Diabetic Cookbook for Beginners," it's important to reflect on our path. This book was not just about recipes; it was about transforming our relationship with food in managing diabetes.

Empowerment Through Knowledge: We started by debunking myths and laying a foundation of understanding about diabetes and nutrition. Knowledge is power; with the information you've gained, you're better equipped to make informed decisions about your diet and health.

The Joy of Cooking and Eating: The recipes and nutritional guidelines are designed to bring joy back to your kitchen and dining table. Remember, managing diabetes doesn't mean sacrificing flavor or enjoyment. It's about finding balance and savoring every bite with mindfulness and appreciation.

A Journey, Not a Destination: Managing diabetes is an ongoing journey. There will be days of success and days of challenge. Embrace each day as an opportunity to nourish your body and soul. Keep experimenting with recipes and flavors, and remember that each meal is a step towards better health.

Community and Support: You are not alone on this journey. Share your experiences, recipes, and learnings with others. Support from family, friends, and fellow diabetics can be incredibly empowering. Together, you can inspire and motivate each other.

Looking Ahead: As you close this book, consider it not an end but a beginning. The beginning of a healthier, more vibrant life where you are in control of your diabetes rather than it controlling you. Keep learning, keep experimenting, and most importantly, enjoy the delicious health and wellness journey.

Thank you for allowing this book to be a part of your journey. May each recipe bring health, happiness, and a sense of accomplishment. Here's to a healthier, happier you!

Appendix A: 30 day Meal Plan

Day	Breakfast (Pg.)	Snack (Pg.)	Lunch (Pg.)	Afternoon Snack (Pg.)	Dinner (Pg.)
1	Oatmeal with Berries and Nuts (22)	Apple Cinnamon Yogurt Parfait (63)	Tuna Salad with Whole Wheat Pita (36)	Roasted Chickpeas (64)	Baked Lemon Garlic Tilapia (49)
2	Scrambled Eggs with Spinach and Whole Wheat Toast (23)	Baked Apple Chips (65)	Chicken and Avocado Lettuce Wraps (37)	Peanut Butter and Banana Roll-Ups (66)	Grilled Chicken and Vegetable Skewers (50)
3	Greek Yogurt with Mixed Berries and Nuts (24)	Cottage Cheese and Fruit Bowl (68)	Vegetable Soup with Quinoa (38)	Vegetable Hummus Dip (69)	Turkey Meatloaf with Sweet Potato Topping (51)
4	Apple Cinnamon Oatmeal Pancakes (25)	Whole Grain Crackers with Cheese and Tomato (70)	Grilled Chicken Salad with Mixed Greens (39)	Mini Veggie Frittatas (71)	Baked Salmon with Roasted Asparagus (52)
5	Turkey and Vegetable Frittata (27)	Classic Baked Apple Crisp (73)	Egg Salad on Whole Wheat Bread (40)	Vanilla Brown Rice Pudding (74)	Vegetarian Stuffed Peppers (54)
6	Banana Walnut Baked Oatmeal (28)	Peach Cobbler with Cinnamon Crust (76)	Broccoli and Cheese Stuffed Baked Potatoes (41)	Lemon Bars with Shortbread Crust (77)	Shrimp and Broccoli Stir-Fry (55)
7	Avocado Toast with Poached Eggs (29)	Old-Fashioned Bread Pudding (78)	Turkey and Cranberry Sandwich (42)	Baked Custard with Nutmeg (79)	Beef and Vegetable Stew (56)
8	Berry Smoothie Bowl (30)	Mixed Berry Compote with Yogurt (80)	Spinach and Feta Cheese Wrap (43)	No-Bake Peanut Butter Oat Bars (81)	Baked Cod with Herb Crust (58)

Day	Breakfast (Pg.)	Snack (Pg.)	Lunch (Pg.)	Afternoon Snack (Pg.)	Dinner (Pg.)
9	Vegetable and Cheese Omelette (31)	Baked Banana Pudding (82)	Roasted Vegetable Quiche (45)	Cinnamon-Spiced Baked Pears (83)	Vegetarian Chili (59)
10	Whole Wheat Blueberry Muffins (32)	Classic Hot Lemon and Honey Tea (86)	Black Bean and Corn Salad (46)	Classic Banana Smoothie (87)	Herb Roasted Chicken with Vegetables (60)
11	Oatmeal with Berries and Nuts (22)	Green Tea with Mint and Honey (88)	Tuna Salad with Whole Wheat Pita (36)	Classic Strawberry Smoothie (89)	Baked Lemon Garlic Tilapia (49)
12	Scrambled Eggs with Spinach and Whole Wheat Toast (23)	Classic Iced Tea with Lemon (90)	Chicken and Avocado Lettuce Wraps (37)	Blueberry Almond Milk Smoothie (91)	Grilled Chicken and Vegetable Skewers (50)
13	Greek Yogurt with Mixed Berries and Nuts (24)	Warm Spiced Apple Cider (92)	Vegetable Soup with Quinoa (38)	Cucumber and Mint Infused Water (93)	Turkey Meatloaf with Sweet Potato Topping (51)
14	Apple Cinnamon Oatmeal Pancakes (25)	Ginger Peach Iced Tea (94)	Grilled Chicken Salad with Mixed Greens (39)	Raspberry Lemonade (95)	Baked Salmon with Roasted Asparagus (52)
15	Turkey and Vegetable Frittata (27)	Classic Tomato Sauce (97)	Egg Salad on Whole Wheat Bread (40)	Honey Mustard Dressing (98)	Vegetarian Stuffed Peppers (54)
16	Banana Walnut Baked Oatmeal (28)	Classic Cranberry Sauce (99)	Broccoli and Cheese Stuffed Baked Potatoes (41)	Garlic Herb Butter (100)	Shrimp and Broccoli Stir-Fry (55)

Day	Breakfast (Pg.)	Snack (Pg.)	Lunch (Pg.)	Afternoon Snack (Pg.)	Dinner (Pg.)
17	Avocado Toast with Poached Eggs (29)	Avocado Cilantro Lime Dressing (101)	Turkey and Cranberry Sandwich (42)	Barbecue Sauce (102)	Beef and Vegetable Stew (56)
18	Berry Smoothie Bowl (30)	Lemon Dill Sauce (103)	Spinach and Feta Cheese Wrap (43)	Caramelized Onion Relish (104)	Baked Cod with Herb Crust (58)
19	Vegetable and Cheese Omelette (31)	Creamy Horseradish Sauce (105)	Roasted Vegetable Quiche (45)	Maple Cinnamon Apple Sauce (106)	Vegetarian Chili (59)
20	Whole Wheat Blueberry Muffins (32)	Roast Turkey with Herb Butter (109)	Black Bean and Corn Salad (46)	Green Bean Casserole (110)	Herb Roasted Chicken with Vegetables (60)
21	Oatmeal with Berries and Nuts (22)	Classic Mashed Potatoes (111)	Tuna Salad with Whole Wheat Pita (36)	Sweet Potato Casserole with Low-Glycemic Topping (112)	Baked Lemon Garlic Tilapia (49)
22	Scrambled Eggs with Spinach and Whole Wheat Toast (23)	Traditional Pumpkin Pie (113)	Chicken and Avocado Lettuce Wraps (37)	Glazed Ham with Pineapple and Cherries (114)	Grilled Chicken and Vegetable Skewers (50)
23	Greek Yogurt with Mixed Berries and Nuts (24)	Herb-Roasted Root Vegetables (115)	Vegetable Soup with Quinoa (38)	Cranberry Orange Relish (116)	Turkey Meatloaf with Sweet Potato Topping (51)
24	Apple Cinnamon Oatmeal Pancakes (25)	Baked Brie and Almonds (117)	Grilled Chicken Salad with Mixed Greens (39)	Eggnog (118)	Baked Salmon with Roasted Asparagus (52)

Day	Breakfast (Pg.)	Snack (Pg.)	Lunch (Pg.)	Afternoon Snack (Pg.)	Dinner (Pg.)
25	Turkey and Vegetable Frittata (27)	Apple Cinnamon Yogurt Parfait (63)	Egg Salad on Whole Wheat Bread (40)	Roasted Chickpeas (64)	Vegetarian Stuffed Peppers (54)
26	Banana Walnut Baked Oatmeal (28)	Baked Apple Chips (65)	Broccoli and Cheese Stuffed Baked Potatoes (41)	Peanut Butter and Banana Roll-Ups (66)	Shrimp and Broccoli Stir-Fry (55)
27	Avocado Toast with Poached Eggs (29)	Cottage Cheese and Fruit Bowl (68)	Turkey and Cranberry Sandwich (42)	Vegetable Hummus Dip (69)	Beef and Vegetable Stew (56)
28	Berry Smoothie Bowl (30)	Whole Grain Crackers with Cheese and Tomato (70)	Spinach and Feta Cheese Wrap (43)	Mini Veggie Frittatas (71)	Baked Cod with Herb Crust (58)
29	Vegetable and Cheese Omelette (31)	Classic Baked Apple Crisp (73)	Roasted Vegetable Quiche (45)	Vanilla Brown Rice Pudding (74)	Vegetarian Chili (59)
30	Whole Wheat Blueberry Muffins (32)	Peach Cobbler with Cinnamon Crust (76)	Black Bean and Corn Salad (46)	Lemon Bars with Shortbread Crust (77)	Herb Roasted Chicken with Vegetables (60)

Author's Note

Thank you for reading this book.

The creation of this work has been a journey filled with challenges, commitment, and dedication, made possible by your interest and support. Every word and concept reflects hours of thorough research and reflection to provide you with work that informs and inspires.

As we end this journey, I ask for one last valuable contribution: a review on Amazon.com. Your words and feedback are essential for my growth as an author and to help other readers discover this book. To leave your review, scan the QR code below, which will take you directly to the book's page on Amazon.

Thank you in advance for taking the time to share your opinion and for your help in bringing this book to a wider audience.

With gratitude,

Ingrid Lamarr

http://bit.ly/diabeticrev